Dear Future Exam Success Story:

Congratulations on your purchase of our study guide. Our goal in writing our study guide was to cover the content on the test, as well as provide insight into typical test taking mistakes and how to overcome them.

Standardized tests are a key component of being successful, which only increases the importance of doing well in the high-pressure high-stakes environment of test day. How well you do on this test will have a significant impact on your future- and we have the research and practical advice to help you execute on test day.

The product you're reading now is designed to exploit weaknesses in the test itself, and help you avoid the most common errors test takers frequently make.

How to use this study guide

We don't want to waste your time. Our study guide is fast-paced and fluff-free. We suggest going through it a number of times, as repetition is an important part of learning new information and concepts.

First, read through the study guide completely to get a feel for the content and organization. Read the general success strategies first, and then proceed to the content sections. Each tip has been carefully selected for its effectiveness.

Second, read through the study guide again, and take notes in the margins and highlight those sections where you may have a particular weakness.

Finally, bring the manual with you on test day and study it before the exam begins.

Your success is our success

We would be delighted to hear about your success. Send us an email and tell us your story. Thanks for your business and we wish you continued success-

Sincerely,

Mometrix Test Preparation Team

Need more help? Check out our flashcards at:
http://MometrixFlashcards.com/ARDMS

TABLE OF CONTENTS

Top 20 Test Taking Tips

1. Carefully follow all the test registration procedures
2. Know the test directions, duration, topics, question types, how many questions
3. Setup a flexible study schedule at least 3-4 weeks before test day
4. Study during the time of day you are most alert, relaxed, and stress free
5. Maximize your learning style; visual learner use visual study aids, auditory learner use auditory study aids
6. Focus on your weakest knowledge base
7. Find a study partner to review with and help clarify questions
8. Practice, practice, practice
9. Get a good night's sleep; don't try to cram the night before the test
10. Eat a well balanced meal
11. Know the exact physical location of the testing site; drive the route to the site prior to test day
12. Bring a set of ear plugs; the testing center could be noisy
13. Wear comfortable, loose fitting, layered clothing to the testing center; prepare for it to be either cold or hot during the test
14. Bring at least 2 current forms of ID to the testing center
15. Arrive to the test early; be prepared to wait and be patient
16. Eliminate the obviously wrong answer choices, then guess the first remaining choice
17. Pace yourself; don't rush, but keep working and move on if you get stuck
18. Maintain a positive attitude even if the test is going poorly
19. Keep your first answer unless you are positive it is wrong
20. Check your work, don't make a careless mistake

Sound

For any medical imaging modality, a fundamental energy unit must be defined. Around this unit, the processes of energy production, interaction with the target, energy reception, and image formation will be carried out. In the case of ultrasound, the fundamental energy unit is the sound wave. Sound is a naturally occurring mechanism that we as humans perceive on a daily basis. It has been harnessed quite ingeniously by ultrasonic devices to produce an image of part of the human body. The understanding of sound and its behavior is the first step in understanding how ultrasound works.

Before sound can be defined, the concept of a medium must first be defined. A medium is simply any large volume of matter; examples of media are air, water, and in the case of ultrasound, body tissue. Each is made up of infinitely many subunits, or "particles," that are perceived to be evenly spaced and motionless relative to each other. The concept of a medium is fairly simple, as humans we are continuously surrounded by a medium of air that contains subunits of nitrogen, hydrogen, and oxygen. However the presence of a medium is critical in ultrasound imaging because sound *requires* a medium, that is sound cannot exist in a vacuum. The properties of a given medium also heavily influence the manner in which sound moves or propagates through it.

A sound wave can be envisioned as an organized series of interruptions. The nature of these "interruptions" is an oscillation in the constituent particles of the medium, causing them to alternately be positioned closer to and farther apart from each other. The oscillations and therefore the sound wave must be produced by a source, will cross its medium in a straight line until a target is reached. A tuning fork is the easiest source to imagine, it physically oscillates back and forth causing adjacent air molecules to oscillate with it.

This movement causes a shift in several physical properties of the medium. The most significant of these is pressure, which undergoes local compression and rarefraction in a regular, alternating pattern. Graphically, pressure as a function of time for a given point in a medium through which sound propagates will appear as a sine wave.

However, recall that the sound wave is not stationary but propagates across its medium; while one area of the medium is compressed, the area ahead of it in the medium becomes rarefracted. For this point, rarefraction must be followed by compression, so the sound wave "moves" one step forward. If we were to set a fixed time and observe a larger section of the entire medium, a graph of pressure with respect to *distance* would also appear as a sine wave.

In combining these two ideas, we see that the true, full appearance of sound is that of a "moving" sine wave. The cause of this movement is the manner in which adjacent points in the medium oscillate at slight offsets to each other. Consider as an example the ripples generated by throwing a rock into a pond. A snapshot of the surface of the water at a given time would reveal a sinusoidal pattern, while a close-up of a single location on the pond extended over a period of time would also reveal a sinusoidal pattern. The overall appearance is of moving waves propagating outwards from the point of contact.

Wave Equation

Several variables are used to visualize and quantify the sound wave, many of which come from standard trigonometry. The two most important in terms of ultrasound are amplitude and frequency. For this application, amplitude is the change in pressure from rest to maximum compression or from rest to maximum rarefraction. Similarly the "cycle" used in calculating frequency is the process of shifting from maximum compression to maximum rarefraction and back to maximum compression; the length of time for this cycle to occur is called the period. Frequency then is calculated as 1/period and is a measure of how "fast" the oscillations occur.

A standard format for expressing these two variables when describing a sound wave is known as the *wave equation.* θ

$$S(t) = A\cos(wt + \theta)\square$$

In this equation, sound is represented by S, as a function of time t; amplitude is represented by A, frequency is represented by $\square$ (generally in radians/sec), and phase is represented by $\square$. Phase will be discussed in the forthcoming section. Note that sound could also be represented as a function of position rather than time.

The audible range for humans is from 20Hz to 20kHz; the greater the frequency of sound wave the higher its pitch will be. Other animals might have a wider audible range, this is why "dog whistles" don't bother us. The term "ultrasound" specifically refers to sound waves above 20kHz and thus above the audible range of humans. In ultrasound imaging the sound waves used to acquire images of the body range typically from 2 - 10Mhz, well outside of our audible range.

Quantitative Properties

In addition to the basic properties of amplitude and frequency, there are several other variables that help to define a sound wave. These variables can be divided into three categories, each of which describe a dimension spanned by sound:

1. **Time**
   <u>Period</u> - *amount of time required for one cycle to pass. Also equal to the inverse of frequency, and measured in seconds.*
   <u>Phase</u> - *amount of offset or delay. This can be expressed with respect to the origin or with respect to another waveform of equal frequency, and is measured as a fraction of the full period.*
2. **Space**
   <u>Speed</u> - *rate at which one point of the waveform (usually the front) progresses through the medium. This is a function of the properties of the medium and is expressed as a distance over time, usually m/s.*
   <u>Wavelength</u> - *similar to the period, but in the spatial domain. The wavelength describes the distance covered by one cycle of the waveform as it progresses through the medium. It is calculated as the speed times the period. Again, period is the* duration *of one oscillation while wavelength is the* length *of one oscillation.*
3. **Magnitude**
   <u>Intensity</u> - *more commonly used instead of amplitude in order to quantify the magnitude of displacement imposed by a sound wave. Intensity is equal to the power carried by the sound wave averaged over a given period of time.*

Power = force x displacement/time

Power = force exerted by pressure wave x medium velocity

Intensity = $\dfrac{Vmax^2}{2Z}$

4. *It represents how "loud" the sound is, and is expressed in decibels.*

The above variables are summarized in the following table:

Variable	Symbol	Unit
Period	T	seconds
Phase	▯	radians
Speed	v	meters/second
Wavelength	▯	meters
Intensity	I	decibels

Pulse-mode

The sound wave has until this point been described as a continuous sine wave, logically this form of ultrasound transmission is known as "continuous-mode". While this description represents sound in its truest and most natural form, an alternate method of sound generation is used more commonly in ultrasound and is known as "pulse-mode" or "pulsed ultrasound." Pulse-mode is preferred over continuous-mode because it takes better advantage of the properties of sound as applied to image formation, and because it simplifies the processes of sound generation and detection.

As the name would indicate, a "pulse" is a short burst of sound containing only a few cycles. A very basic pulse could be generated by turning your stereo on and then off very quickly. In pulse-mode ultrasound, the transducer is triggered such that it generates pulses of sound at set time intervals. The mechanisms of generation and means of quantification of the sound wave are fundamentally the same, except that the "down time" in between pulses must be factored in. Each pulse itself is made up of several sound waves, each of different frequency, superimposed upon each other and lasting for only a few cycles; the multiple-frequency composition allows the pulse to carry more information than would a single-frequency pulse when it comes time to reconstruct the received image.

In analyzing the entire signal that is output from the transducer, each pulse is viewed as a single, discrete unit. Rather than treating one full cycle of the continuous sine wave as an "event" as in the case of continuous-mode ultrasound, we now treat one pulse as an "event." Thus the same quantifiers used to describe the oscillations in continuous mode are translated to describe the pulses in pulsed-mode. For example:

1. Pulse repetition frequency - The number of pulses that occur in one second.
2. Pulse repetition period - The amount of time in between pulses, that is the duration of the pulse itself plus the duration of the ensuing quiet period.
3. Pulse duration - The length of time required for only the pulse itself to be transmitted.
4. Duty factor - The fraction of "noisy time" to "quiet time", or pulse duration divided by pulse repetition period.

The purpose of pulse-mode will become clearer as we examine the interaction of sound with its surrounding medium and the methods by which transmitted sound is used to construct an image. The benefits of having discrete, separable bursts of sound rather than a single continuous signal will then become more apparent.

Mechanisms of Sound Generation

The physical generation of sound requires the displacement of particles that comprise the surrounding medium back and forth in order to generate the previously described waveform in an adjustable manner. Such an activity requires a device known as a transducer. In the case of ultrasound wave generation the initial form of energy used by the transducer is a controlled electrical voltage, and the final form of energy is mechanical movement. This is a unique form of transduction; materials that can perform it are termed piezoelectric. Piezoelectricity can occur naturally in certain substances; most commonly, quartz crystals exist having an electrical construction that causes reshaping when an external voltage is applied. This reshaping pushes the air molecules surrounding the crystals in such a manner that sound is produced. Other piezoelectric elements have been artificially produced via the polarization of a ferroelectric material followed by heating and then slow cooling in the presence of an electric field; these are known as polarized ferroelectrics. Both natural and artificial piezoelectric elements use electric dipoles in their construction that realign under the presence of an applied voltage, causing the element to reshape.

The piezoelectric crystals used in ultrasound are flat and circular in shape and vibrate at a natural resonant frequency when electrically stimulated. That is, applying a voltage of varying magnitude will cause a sound of varying intensity to be produced, however this sound will be of a set frequency. Resonant frequency is inversely proportional to crystal thickness, therefore in order to change the frequency of the sound generated, a piezoelectric crystal of different thickness must be used. Transducers may be manipulated in ultrasound in many different ways in order to control their effects, for example while a single piezoelectric crystal makes up a *single-element transducer*, several crystals can be joined together to form a *multiple-element transducer*. The benefits of using multiple elements will be later explored.

While the piezoelectric crystal makes up the heart of the transducer, several other elements must also be included to ensure proper function. As we will see, the air-tissue interface in front of the face of the transducer will cause much of the transmitted energy from the piezoelectric element to be reflected back at the transducer, therefore a matching layer is used to mimic the properties of tissue and reduce or eliminate this interface. Backing material is used to reduce unwanted vibration, echoes, or backwardly-transmitted sound that would cause noise in the transducer. Especially in the case of pulse-mode ultrasound, the transducer must be able to generate short, distinct sound waves. The backing material essentially allows it to turn on and off quickly, without any lingering vibration. These elements are all contained within the transducer housing. External connections allow electrical stimulation of the electrodes, which of course cause movement of the piezoelectric crystal, ultimately resulting in the generation of sound.

Beam Formation

While a sound wave comprises a single straight line of activity that moves through its medium, in Ultrasound practice many sound waves are used together, encompassing a certain thickness called a "beam." Similar to the light of a flashlight, a sound beam can be visualized as the region in front of the transducer that can receive or "hear" the sound wave, within which objects can be imaged. Immediately in front of the transducer, this region would have the shape of the transducer face; at farther depths the profile changes significantly. The shape of the beam is highly dependent on properties of its transducer; specifically the two properties that affect beam profile are radius and resonant frequency. Resonant frequency is a function of the transducer's thickness, thus the "output" can be completely controlled by the physical dimensions of the piezoelectric crystal.

The behavior of the ultrasound beam obeys Huygens' Principle, that is the beam generated by the entire source (transducer) may be considered as the sum of the beams generated by an infinite number of point sources. In the case of sound, each point source generates sound equally in all directions creating a spherical wave. The summation of these spherical waves forms the beam profile.

As you can see, the beam initially converges, in a region called the near field, and then diverges through the region known as the far field, up to infinity. These two regions are quantified as follows

Near Field Length (NFL) = $\dfrac{a^2}{\lambda}$

Far Field Divergence Angle = (θ)

$\square = \sin^{-1} \dfrac{(.61 \times \lambda)}{a}$

where a is the radius of the transducer. Recall that λ, or wavelength, is a function of the speed of sound in the medium - a constant - and transducer frequency. Adjustment either of the two major quantifiers - radius or frequency - will allow for full control over the beam profile. While a single-element transducer of course cannot change its diameter, a multiple-element transducer can effectively do so by turning on or off the elements around its perimeter. An increase in diameter will cause an increase in the length of the near field and a decrease in the angle of divergence throughout the far field; these dimensions factor into the lateral resolution and focusing of the device.

The convergence angle of the near field is controlled by a lens placed in front of the transducer, which serves to focus the beam. Without a lens, sound would propagate outwards equally in all directions, rendering the transducer useless in terms of ultrasound. However, with a concave acoustic lens, the individual sound beams are deflected inwards throughout the Near Field Length. The cause of the beam's divergence at the end of the near field is unknown, however the result is that the beam thickness is at a minimum at medium distances, an area called the focal region. This region is the optimum length for obtaining an image from the sound wave, thus techniques are used by ultrasound designers to allow adjustment of the focal region onto the area of interest.

In addition to a piezoelectric crystal and an acoustic lens, the transducer contains two other elements that aid in maximizing its efficiency at generating a pure sound beam to be used in imaging the body. The first is a backing element, which is placed on the side of the transducer across from the beam to be generated. The purpose of the backing element is to absorb vibration from the transducer and remove any sound directed backwards, as these serve no useful purpose. The second item is a matching layer, which is placed in front of the piezoelectric crystal on the side of the beam. Its purpose is to serve as an intermediary between the surface of the piezoelectric element and the surface to be imaged; as we will see the drastically different properties of these two surfaces could cause problems without this intermediary.

Phase Steering

As the mechanics of the transducer can be manipulated to alter the dimensions of the sound beam, they can also be manipulated to alter the *direction* of the sound beam or beams. By using a multiple-element transducer, the time delay or phase offset of the various sound waves can be adapted such that the beam profiles generated by the transducer match a given application. For example, taking into account Huygens' Principle, consider a linear array in which each piezoelectric element sitting next in line is electrically stimulated after an appropriate delay. The net effect, as you can see, is a steered beam that leaves the transducer at an angle. Or, the same linear array can be fired such that the outer elements are stimulated before the inner elements, leading to a focused beam. The phase offset of multiple element transducers is one more variable that can be manipulated in the refinement of the ultrasound beam towards a specific application.

Sound Propagation/Interaction with Target

Effects of Medium/Tissue

At the start of image acquisition sound is produced by a transducer, introduced into a medium, and allowed to propagate. The events that occur during this period of propagation are functions of the target medium and its components but are fairly predictable. If the medium is a bucket of water, the sound wave will propagate in a straightforward manner at a constant speed and direction; its properties will change very little with distance as the medium is uniform. However in ultrasound applications the medium in question is the human body, which is very non-uniform and contains multiple elements. As a result, the projected sound wave will interact with the target medium in various haphazard yet calculable ways, ultimately a return signal or signals will end up back at the transducer. The principle interactions that take place between the sound wave and its medium are classified as attenuation and reflection, both of which can be demonstrated by the simple example of standing across a football field from a friend and having him or her shout at you. Two effects will be recognized: first, the farther away your friend is, the harder it will be to hear him -- attenuation. Second an echo can be heard very shortly after the initial shout -- reflection.

Attenuation

The first of these effects is known as attenuation, an event that occurs in every medium (in the above example, the medium is air). Simply put, the intensity of a sound wave decreases with distance. As sound propagates, the particle oscillations that it causes require energy, causing the wave to lose energy mostly in the form of heat. The wave's intensity is a unitless quantity that is often taken to be unity at the transducer; because intensity only decreases at any point afterward it can be compared fractionally to its initial value. When expressed in decibels (further explained below), the rate of attenuation becomes a linear function, that is each time the sound wave covers a certain distance, a set amount of decrease in intensity will occur. This relationship does not change within the medium, it is a property specific to each different type of medium and is quantified by a variable called the attenuation coefficient. The larger the attenuation coefficient, the more rapidly the intensity of the sound wave will decrease. Air has a relatively small attenuation coefficient, which is why you would still hear your friend at the other end of a football field (a relatively large distance). Water, conversely, has a high attenuation coefficient. If your same friend was shouting at you underwater in a large pool, you would have a harder time hearing. As a general rule of thumb, a value of 1 dB per cm per MHz is used to define the attenuation of an ultrasound in soft tissue.

Reflection

The second effect demonstrated in the example, the echo, is a result of a phenomenon known as reflection. Reflection too is an easily understood event that requires two adjacent media in which sound propagates. Reflection occurs at the interface between the two media with the amount of reflection depending on the acoustic impedance of the two media. Impedance is a difficult property to comprehend, mathematically it is equal to the product of two other material properties: density, which is the weight per given volume, and acoustic velocity, which specifies the speed at which sound naturally propagates through the material.

Impedance = density x velocity

Impedance is equal to a resistance to movement, however this has an inverse effect on the sound wave. Materials with a higher acoustic impedance will allow sound to pass through faster. Since acoustic velocity is a set property and is nearly the same for all biological tissue (with bone being an exception), impedance is essentially directly proportional to density.

Now that impedance has been (loosely) defined, the process of reflection can be examined within the context of an ultrasound wave propagating through body tissue. Reflection of sound in a medium is exactly what the name would imply - upon striking an interface, a sound wave will "bounce" back and propagate in the opposite direction.

An interface therefore is defined as the surface joining two adjacent mediums having different impedance values. It acts much like a wall that causes thrown tennis balls to bounce off of it. In fact, most interfaces within the body are caused by the walls of tissue or organs whose impedances differ from their surroundings. However, upon reaching a typical interface the sound wave will not be reflected entirely, only a fraction of it will bounce back while the remainder will continue to pass in the original direction and into the second medium. The two partial sound waves will have decreased pressure amplitude relative to the initial sound wave.

dB notation

Unlike frequency, which is a numerically calculable and measurable quantity, the magnitude of the sound wave is essentially a unitless term. While it is possible to measure the degree of displacement of particles created by a given sound wave, the general convention used instead is to define some level of magnitude as a standard unit and to relate any other given magnitude as a fraction of this standard unit. In practice, these fractional terms can span a range of exponential proportions, so the decibel format is used.

One decibel is an arbitrary magnitude that has been chosen as the standard, base unit for sound and incorporated into everyday use. For example, the volume of a person whispering is equal to 30dB, the volume of a normal conversation stands at around 60dB, while the volume of a jet plane launching represents 130dB. In the case of ultrasound, however, volume (i.e. magnitude) is generated at an initial level and then *decreases* from there on. The same relationship will apply, only that each new magnitude X expressed in dB will now be a negative term due to the fact that the fraction X/S is less than one.

In addition to simplicity of terms, another advantage of using the decibel format in ultrasound is the compression of the integer range or expansion of the fractional range. The magnitude of sound covers an enormous dynamic range. Use of the decibel format shrinks this to a more manageable range; for example the difference between 1dB and 100dB is a factor of 100,000. The opposite is true of the fractional range; an extremely small dynamic range is expanded by using the decibel convention.

Refraction

We have described how a sound wave will reflect off of a flat, perpendicular interface back towards its origin. Unfortunately, the majority of surfaces encountered in the body do not meet these criteria, that is, they are irregularly shaped and oddly positioned, which of course causes some complications. First consider a sound wave striking a non-perpendicular surface/interface, i.e. striking a flat interface at a given angle of incidence. Much like a pool ball striking a rail, this incident beam will be reflected away from the surface at an angle equal to its angle of incidence, away from the normal line. The departure angle, or angle of reflection, is equal to the angle of incidence. As in the case of a perpendicular incident beam, the reflected beam represents a fraction of the incident beam while the remainder, or transmitted beam, continues in its original direction. The transmitted beam simultaneously undergoes another process known as refraction. Refraction is caused by the differential impedance across the interface. As the sound beam, which spans a certain width, strikes this interface at a non-perpendicular angle it is slowed at a rate not uniform across its width, causing redirection. The same phenomenon can be observed by sticking a spear into a bucket of water: the spear appears to enter the water at a certain angle, then continue through underneath the water at a different angle. The spear does not actually bend, but the light waves that are perceived by the eye do, again caused by the change in impedance. While the reflected beam travels at an angle θ_r that is equal to the incident angle θ_i, the angle of the transmitted beam θ_t relates to the incident angle in a manner proportionate to the acoustic velocity of the two mediums. This behavior is governed by a set of equations similar to that of simple perpendicular reflection, with the angles accounted for. However, due to an interesting phenomenon, for an incident beam approaching above a critical angle θ_{ic}, complete reflection will occur.

Scatter

Again we must shift our attention from the ideal to the real in order to introduce a phenomenon present in ultrasound. No medium in the body is completely homogenous, and no surface is completely flat. Both of these properties lead to scatter, which occurs when small imperfections cause seemingly random reflections and refractions of the sound wave in all directions. This can exist in two forms: rough surfaces at impedance boundaries or suspended particles in the medium. Scatter is caused by *small* imperfections; small by definition is a term relative to the wavelength of the sound beam. Since a higher frequency waveform has a smaller wavelength, the imperfections in the surrounding medium will be larger relative to it, and it will be subject to a larger amount of scatter. In addition to frequency, the amount of scatter that will occur is dependent on the number of scatterers, the average size of the scatterers, and the amount of impedance difference between the scatterers and its surrounding or adjacent medium. While these imperfections do not greatly degrade the properties of the sound beam, their effects are significant enough to warrant mention.

Single Line Reconstruction

As has been described, a sound wave pulse projected into a medium will partially reflect back towards its generating transducer upon striking any interface within the medium. These interfaces generally occur at boundaries between different tissue types being imaged. The job of the transducer is not only to generate the initial sound pulse but to subsequently listen for reflected sound pulses striking its surface. Upon "hearing" the echoes, it must convert these pulses into electrical signals that are later reconstructed to form an image. Reflected pulses are the backbone of ultrasound: when an ultrasound image is displayed it is the *interfaces* that serve as data points to be visualized. To understand how a received sequence of echo pulses is used to reconstruct a complete image outlining the layout of tissue within the body, it is easiest to first consider a single one-dimensional strip of medium, which conceptually represents the area covered by a single sound wave.

The multiple interfaces in the path of the transducer and the sound pulse it generates will create a received signal consisting of a series of reflected pulses, or echoes. These echoes can be graphed with respect to time as shown below:

An echo is defined by two pieces of information: time and magnitude. Each is relative to the transmitted pulse at the transducer: time represents the duration of the period beginning at initial sound pulse generation, continuing through its reflection by a given interface, and finally concluding at its reception back at the transducer. Since there are multiple interfaces off of which the transmitted beam can reflect, multiple echoes will result from a single transmitted pulse. Magnitude represents the intensity of the received echo pulse as a fraction of the intensity of the initial sound pulse. Time and magnitude data are used together to back-calculate information about the interfaces that caused each echo. First, time can be translated into the distance from transducer to interface. Such a relationship depends simply on the acoustic velocity of the medium; assuming this to be constant, a time-distance proportionality is now defined. Second, the magnitude of the echo indicates the degree of impedance mismatch on either side of the interface. Larger impedance mismatches cause a larger fraction of the transmitted sound pulse to be reflected, and therefore cause a larger echo. Since the surrounding medium is usually assumed to be that of known impedance (i.e. water), when the amount of impedance mismatch is known the impedance of the tissue across the first interface encountered can be calculated. At each ensuing interface downstream, the same information is known and therefore the impedance of each forthcoming tissue can be determined.

Once the location of each interface is known and the impedance values of the tissues on either side of each interface is also known, an image can be constructed. Because we are considering only the area imaged by a single sound wave, our resulting image will consist of a one-dimensional "strip" of data.

Throughout this strip, the distance to each interface will of course translate into a distance along the representative image. The magnitude of the impedance mismatch at each interface can be directly graphed (a format known as A-mode) but is more commonly translated to a brightness level in the image (B-mode). The sample data acquired above represents a one-dimensional region of tissue and therefore produces a one-dimensional image, as shown:

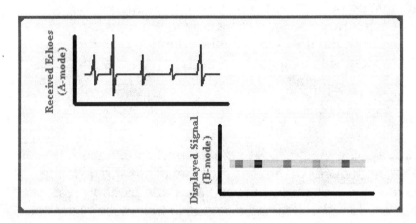

Multiple Line Reconstruction

The algorithm used in single-line reconstruction forms the backbone of ultrasound imaging; a two-dimensional image can easily be reconstructed by repeating many times the procedure for reconstructing a single line. Beginning on one edge of the area of interest, the transducer is swept across the region, acquiring one-dimensional images as described above at set spatial intervals. If each line of data is taken close enough to its adjacent line, then a complete image will be formed.

Two constraints should be noted. First, one entire line of data must be acquired before the next can be initiated. This is due to the fact that the same transducer is used for both generating the transmitted pulse and receiving the reflected echoes. Second, the entire image must be acquired and updated quickly enough that it can be perceived in real-time. The human eye works at a "speed" of 30 frames per second, therefore the entire ultrasound image must be acquired in 1/30 sec, or about 30ms. These two constraints limit how much information can be acquired since ultimately sound only travels so fast. Using a whole row of transducers rather than one transducer that repositions itself will speed up the acquisition to a large degree, but this adds physical as well as computational complexity. The temporal limitation on the depth and number of lines that can be received therefore limits the quality or resolution of the formed image.

Another geometry for acquiring multiple lines of data is the sector scan. In this format, a single transducer is again used but rather than moving it along an edge to acquire each new line, it is pivoted about a single point. This results in the familiar pie-shaped image that is most commonly seen in ultrasound. Mechanically the sector scan is much more precise and reliable than the linear-array scan.

Calculations

The first calculation that must be performed in constructing an image from received ultrasonic data is converting the amount of time to the reception of an echo pulse into the distance from the transducer to the interface that generated that pulse. The key to this relationship is acoustic velocity, which is a constant rate of distance over time. By rearranging terms we get:

Distance = velocity x time

In our case, the sound wave pulse must travel to the interface, then upon reflection travel back to the transducer before it is received. Thus the distance covered is actually *twice* the actual distance between the transducer and the interface, so the more correct equation defining distance to transducer would be:

Distance = ½ x velocity x time

In using this relationship, we must assume that acoustic velocity remains constant. In fact there may be minor differences in the speed of sound through various tissue types, however they are taken to be small enough to assume an average for soft tissue, 1540 m/s, as a general value. The one exception for this is the acoustic velocity of *air*, which is much lower than that of soft tissue. Special calculations may need to be made when imaging the lung or any region containing air bubbles. Once distance to the transducer has been calculated, this value is converted into a distance across the visible screen by means highly specific to the image display device.

Sound Detection/Image Formation

Swept Gain Control

As sound travels through a uniform medium, it does not maintain a constant intensity but is attenuated at a constant rate. This property must be taken into account when reconstructing an ultrasound image. This is again a simple calculation based on assumed known properties of the medium: given an average attenuation coefficient, the received pulses can be "regrown" or amplified to their proper intensity based on their distance from the transducer (which has already been determined.) Since amplification per distance is a constant function, the visual appearance of the correction factor is a ramp function that realigns the received pulses, such that echoes from interfaces that are farther away are amplified by a greater amount. This is sometimes referred to as swept-gain control, or time-gain control.

Mechanisms of Reception

A transducer element converts a received ultrasound signal into an electrical stimulus; the means by which it does this is simply the reverse of how it generates sound from electronic input. In this case, the piezoelectric crystals respond to a mechanical deformation caused by sound by producing an electrical current. The magnitude of this output is proportional to the degree of deformation of the crystal, which translates to the amount of oscillation in pressure or the intensity of the incoming sound. The greater the sound wave, the greater the electrical output.

Since ultrasound signals are usually transmitted and received in pulse-mode, the process is simplified in that the transducer receives separate, discrete pulses of data rather than a continuous stream of information. Each echo pulse is separable and can be stored digitally in both the time and magnitude domains, that is the signal can be represented by a sequence of discrete values. Once the sound wave has been converted into this digital signal, it can be computationally analyzed, stored, and otherwise processed by computer in order to ultimately produce an image.

Applications and Techniques

Implementation

With the underlying principles in place, the next step in the development of ultrasound is to put together a device to implement these ideas. As will be explained below, an ultrasound machine contains four basic parts: a pulser, a receiver, a memory/processing unit, and a display. These parts work together to generate the transmitted sound wave pulse, receive the echoes returning from the medium, calculate from these echoes the underlying tissue structure, and display a graphical representation of this structure to the user. This process repeats itself to continuously update in real time, while a console serves as a means of adapting the device to the specific needs of the user for a given application and affects all four parts.

The job of the <u>pulser</u> is to generate discrete electrical impulse signals at a fixed rate, each of which causes the transducer to generate an ultrasound pulse. The pulser controls both the rate at which electrical and therefore ultrasound pulses are generated (the pulse repetition frequency, or prf) and the magnitude of these pulses. Like the prf, the magnitude of the ultrasound pulses is directly proportional to the magnitude of the pulser's output signal. Larger magnitude ultrasound pulses allow greater sensitivity (that is they allow fractionally smaller echo signals to be detected) but must not exceed certain limits for safety reasons.

During the "quiet" time in between pulses being generated, the ultrasound machine "listens" for echoes returning to the transducer. This is done by the <u>receiver</u>, which accepts electrical pulses directly from the transducer and performs several preprocessing functions before passing the signal on to the central memory/processing unit:

1. <u>Amplification</u> - *Because the initial transmitted pulse is subjected to a large amount of attenuation before eventually returning to the transducer, the magnitudes of the received echoes are generally very small. In order to be interpreted as a more manageable signal to be mapped to a visible brightness range the echoes are amplified. The ratio of amplification, a constant by which the input signal is multiplied, is referred to as the* gain *of the receiver and is usually expressed in dB.*
2. <u>Compensation</u> - *The degree of attenuation of the transmitted signal is a function of distance, therefore echoes generated by elements that are farther away from the transducer must be amplified to a greater degree than echoes generated by closer elements in order to restore each to their proper magnitude. Compensation is the application of swept-gain control to perform this correction.*

3. Compression - *Again considering the effects of attenuation, the high amount of signal loss that could occur depending on the position of the sound wave reflectors, causes a large amount of variation in the range of received echo pulses. That is in one case all of the received echoes could be of similar magnitude, while in the next case they could all be of very different magnitude. This necessitates* compression, *which is the standardization of the difference between the maximum and minimum received amplitudes, also called the* dynamic range. *Many different formulas exist for shrinking the dynamic range, such as a linear division or a* logarithmic compression, *in which the log of the magnitude of each echo is used. Conversely, the dynamic range could be expanded by using an exponential expansion.*

4. Filtering - *This process takes advantage of the fact that the ultrasound pulses that are transmitted, and therefore the echo pulses that are received, contain signals of specific, known frequency content. The receiver can eliminate unwanted noise by removing any information that is not contained within the correct frequency range and therefore improve the quality and accuracy of the signal.*

5. Rejection - *Another means of removing unwanted signals that do not originate from known sources, rejection is simply the process of eliminating any pulses whose magnitude falls below a certain threshold. While this may cause some "good" data to be lost, the more dominant effect is decreased noise.*

6. Demodulation - *A type of transduction that converts the voltage signal representing echoes to a signal in another format more appropriate for display, such as video. This signal is then passed to the* memory/processing unit.

As the memory/processing unit accepts the end signal from the receiver, its task is to convert the continuous data stream into freezable images, or "frames," which are constantly updated in real time. Recall that the echo pulses at the receiver represent the interfaces of a two-dimensional space mapped to a one-dimensional, time-dependent signal. The means of mapping are based on information such as the layout of the scan lines (linear or sector), the space between scan lines, and the depth of each scan line. The memory/processing unit must deconstruct this data - it must map the sequence of echoes back to a two-dimensional image. This process is referred to as "digital scan conversion," as each scan line in digital format is converted into a section of a viewable image to be displayed. A basic visualization of this procedure for a linear scan can be formed by a checkerboard-type grid whose boxes need to be filled in. Each "box" contains data and is referred to as a pixel, which effectively represents a square region of imaged tissue. The memory/processing unit is given a sequence of digital values representing echo magnitudes and correctly maps them to the two-dimensional grid, most commonly by sweeping across horizontally, filling in pixel value brightnesses by echo magnitudes, and then moving down to the next line. For sector scans, the geometry is slightly different but the principle of image reconstruction remains the same.

The "memory" aspect of this unit involves the division of the data stream into frames. Each frame represents a single "pass" through the imaged field and is quantified by a set length of time on the data stream. The memory unit is so named because it serves the purpose of freezing each entire image while the next one is being constructed. Therefore an entire grid of values forming an image is updated at once as new pixel values enter the data stream. When this update occurs fast enough to show instantaneous changes in the object being imaged, it is said to be in "real-time."

Any manipulation of data that occurs after the complete image is stored into the memory unit is called post-processing. The most important manipulation that is performed is assigning a brightness level to each digital value stored at the pixel locations. Other post-processing algorithms can be implemented depending on the data that is received.

Finally, the image information stored in memory is useless unless it can be visualized; this is carried out by the display. A wide range of devices can serve as a display - television, computer monitor, digital or analog. The only requirement is that it allow variable brightness levels at each pixel location in order to form an image from memory while updating rapidly enough to maintain real-time motion.

These four components - pulser, receiver, memory/processing unit, and display - work together to form the core of the ultrasound machine. The use of an ultrasound machine to perform diagnostic scans is a complex procedure that is aided by an understanding of each of these components, but nevertheless requires years of clinical experience.

Doppler

Doppler is a specialized application of ultrasound used to image areas that move continuously, or flow. Within the body, this specifically pertains to blood circulating throughout the vasculature. The principle behind Doppler is that for a source that provides an acoustic output of set frequency and a receiver that listens to this output, if either the source or the output is set in motion the frequency at the receiver will change. The basis of this change in frequency is an elongation or shrinking in the time domain of the transmitted sound wave as its source and receiver move away from or towards each other. Each point along its oscillation is set in motion creating a new frequency. In the example on the left the source moves from point A to point B, while in the example on the right the receiver moves from point A to point B. In both cases a "Doppler shift" will occur, the same principle by which radar waves are used by law enforcement officers to obtain vehicle speeds.

In ultrasound, the physical setup of Doppler imaging is the same as in standard ultrasound: a sound wave is transmitted by a source, reflected off of a target, then received back at the source (note that the same physical device, the transducer, acts as both source and receiver.) Because the target is a moving fluid such as blood, the reflected beam effectively comes from a moving source, and it is perceived back at the transducer as having changed in frequency.

A familiar example will confirm this result: when driving a car through a heavy rainstorm, the faster you drive the more quickly the raindrops will appear to come at you. However, in reality they are still falling at the same rate, it is the moving reference point that causes their approach, or "frequency," to change. This is essentially the same as the Doppler effect in which the source (raindrops) is stationary in relation to a moving receiver (car). As an acoustic example, consider the noise of a plane approaching overhead and then flying by. Although the sound emitted by the plane is of a set frequency, its pitch - which is related to frequency - changes as the plane flies by due to the fact that your ears represent a stationary receiver to a moving source.

No matter what the application, the Doppler effect requires a source and a target, at least one of which moves in relation to each other. Ultrasound devices are able to harness the Doppler effect to create a device that uses this frequency change to determine information about blood flow; the difference between the frequency of the transmitted signal and the frequency of the received signal is called the Doppler frequency and is used to calculate the velocity and direction of the blood flow relative to the transducer.

The basic setup for using a Doppler shift to calculate reflector velocity is as shown. A sound beam is transmitted at frequency f_o from the transducer, which reflects off of the moving fluid. The reflectors therefore act as a source that transmits a reflected beam at the same frequency f_o, but since they are in motion the perceived frequency at the transducer is a different frequency f_r. The Doppler frequency f_d is defined as the difference between these two. Clearly when the fluid is moving away from the transducer as in this case, the received frequency f_r will be less than f_o, the velocity of the reflectors is in a sense "subtracted" from the velocity of the oscillations of the sound wave.

$$f_d = f_o - f_r$$

Next, this Doppler frequency is used to calculate the velocity of the moving fluid by another equation that defines Doppler frequency in terms of initial frequency, reflector velocity (V) and the speed of sound (c):

$$v = \frac{f_d \times c}{2f_o}$$

Hardware Controls

While the layout and appearance of ultrasound devices can vary based on manufacturer and model, several universal console elements allow control over the most common processes and settings. The first and most important setting is transducer frequency, which affects a number of characteristics of the image acquisition including beam formation, scatter, and attenuation. Since each piezoelectric element has its own operating frequency, a different physical transducer must be used for each desired beam frequency. Another common feature, pulse repetition frequency, is more readily adjustable by simply altering the rate of electrical stimuli to the pulser; this value is adjusted in order to change the maximum depth that can be imaged.

Turning our attention closer to the signal, the properties of the individual pulse waveforms can be adjusted in order to improve axial resolution. As the duration of the pulse is increased, a larger (worse) axial resolution results. Since each pulse generated by the transducer is a result of a single stimulus from the pulser, the system has no direct means of controlling pulse duration other than changing the physics of the transducer element. Instead, pulse duration is controlled by the amount of damping applied to the pulse after generation. Damping is caused by backing material and/or matching layers and so it is these elements that are influenced by console elements governing pulse duration.

Adjustment of swept-gain is vital to producing an accurate image. The actual controls usually consist of a set of sliding knobs, each mapped to a set distance. The standard setting would be linear, that is greater distances receiving greater amplification, however other layouts may prove more effective after a trial-and-error adjustment period. For example the existence of bone at a certain depth would cause a large amount of attenuation, therefore the region past it would require greater amplification. Most commonly, the barrier between the imaged tissue and the exterior causes a disruption in the linear attenuation slope.

The display unit has a number of controls that act independently of the image acquisition process but nonetheless affect the end result. These are dependent on the unit and include common settings such as brightness, contrast, etc.

Many other processing algorithms can be put under control of the user. Some of the more standard ones have already been mentioned - rejection, compression (logarithmic vs. linear) - while many others have recently been or are being developed. Each machine and each manufacturer will implement its own preprocessing and postprocessing algorithms, some specific to a given application, to create what the designers believe to be the most detailed and most accurate image.

Coupling Gel

One of the first things you'll notice as a patient if you have an ultrasound performed is the application of coupling gel around the area being imaged. The reason this gel is required comes down to the fundamental properties of sound propagation that we have studied: recall that reflection of the sound occurs at impedance boundaries and is a function of the difference in impedance on either side of these boundaries. Also recall that air is a medium having one of the lowest impedances to sound. Putting these two pieces of information together, it is clear that if the face of the transducer that generates the sound wave does not make continuous contact with the skin that overlays the bodily tissue to be imaged, the impending air-tissue interface will preclude any sound propagation from occurring through the body.

The purpose of the coupling gel, therefore, is to remove the air boundary and to allow the transducer-skin interface to maintain as constant an impedance as possible, thus preventing reflection from occurring in this region. The impedance of the coupling gel should be as close as possible to that of the skin surface. Also note that the inner workings of the transducer itself must contain a matching layer such that as sound is generated from its piezoelectric crystal and propagated out its face, the impedance of the material through which it flows matches that of the coupling gel and the bodily tissue.

New Modes

A rapidly developing innovation in ultrasound imaging is that of three-dimensional ultrasound. This process uses a variety of different techniques to acquire a visualized projection of a 3-D volume onto a 2-D image, allowing more information and detail than a standard two-dimensional linear or sector scan. The process of obtaining this volume of data is an extension of the same principles used in 2-D ultrasound with the added steps of sending and receiving sound pulses in multiple planes. Each time this is done, the system must recognize the location of the transducer and direction of the sound beam in order to reconstruct the 3-D volume. The exact physics of how this is done depends on the particular system and application. Because this process takes more time than a 2-D acquisition, movement of the patient becomes and issue, and real-time updates are more difficult to achieve. Various coding or compressional techniques may need to be used.

Contrast agents are used in ultrasound in a fashion similar to those used in radiology. The agent is injected into the bloodstream prior to an image acquisition. When viewing the resulting ultrasound image, the contrast agent stands out against its background, therefore emphasizing the bloodstream and vasculature. This process is frequently used in cardiology in order to image the heart. For the purpose of ultrasound, the contrast agent must have a high reflection coefficient in order to stand out in the image. As we know, air presents the highest impedance mismatch to soft tissue. Therefore, ultrasound contrast agents typically utilize microscopic air bubbles to produce a fluid that reflects sound to a high degree and will be easily visible within the acquired image. Of course, the agent must also be safe for the patient and be cleared from the body in due time.

Another new development in ultrasound is known as Native Tissue Harmonic Imaging (NTHI). To summarize, the property that is utilized in NTHI is the fact that when directing an ultrasound beam into the body, the echoes that return have components not only at the fundamental frequency of the transmitted beam, as previously described, but also at frequencies of integer multiples of this fundamental frequency. For example, if a 2MHz sound wave is transmitted into the body, echoes will return to the transducer having components at frequencies of 2MHz, 4MHz, 6MHz, 8MHz, etc. (These integer multiples are known as the harmonic frequencies in this case). The reason for these harmonic-frequency components is the change in acoustic velocity that occurs as the propagating medium is alternately compressed and relaxed by the sound wave. At each increasing harmonic frequency, the magnitude of the corresponding component of the received echo decreases in magnitude: the majority of information will be contained at the fundamental frequency, the first harmonic (at 4MHz in the example above) will have a lower magnitude, the second harmonic will have a lower magnitude still, and so forth. When transmitting and receiving an ultrasound wave, a large portion of the artifacts/noise that are present are caused by the exterior body wall and are carried only at the fundamental frequency. Therefore, the process of NTHI involves filtering the received echo signal in such a manner as to remove the components that are at the fundamental frequency, leaving only the components at the harmonic frequencies. The result is an improved signal-to-noise ratio and a sharper image.

Safety

As in all imaging procedures, safety to the patient and to the operator are of primary concern. A major benefit of ultrasound is its lack of damaging energy common to xray-based modalities. For this reason, ultrasound is the imaging technique of choice for fetal imaging. Of course, ultrasound waves of sufficient magnitude and/or frequency would be capable of causing damage to body tissue, therefore the operation of ultrasound devices must be governed by predetermined acceptable limits. Clinical trials to determine these levels have been somewhat inconclusive. The impact of sound waves on tissue appear to be largely dependent on the particular tissue being imaged. Nevertheless all data does support that waves of less than 100mW/cm^2 have no damaging bioeffects and are therefore considered safe.

A secondary effect of the transmission of ultrasonic waves into the body is known as cavitation. A rapid decrease in surrounding pressure induced by the sound wave causes bubbles in the medium to expand; subsequent increase in surrounding pressure causes the same bubbles to collapse as well as to increase in internal pressure and in temperature. This increase in temperature may cause serious biological effects, to say nothing of the damaging effects of air bubbles on the quality of the acquired ultrasound image. This process is known as transient cavitation and occurs at high sound wave intensities. At lower intensities, stable cavitation occurs; here the bubbles do not completely collapse. Cavitation can be minimized by removing gas from the imaged medium, by applying external pressure to the medium, by using a higher frequency sound wave, or most simply by using a lower intensity sound wave.

Image Features

The fundamental principles that underlie the generation of an ultrasound image are well defined and under ideal circumstances will allow an exact image representation of a solid medium with perfect features. When applied to the human body, which is extremely non-ideal, many of these fundamentals break down, or at least begin to behave in an unanticipated manner, resulting in an image whose features contain artifacts that must be interpreted properly to gain a correct evaluation of the imaged tissue. By understanding how these fundamentals act imperfectly and recognizing common image features and artifacts, a more correct evaluation can be made.

Scatterers

The most noticeable feature of displayed ultrasound images is the fuzzy or grainy texture about the entire image. This is due to a process known as scatter, which was introduced in section 2. Because each scatterer is small relative to the tissue being imaged, the propagating sound wave as a whole remains intact, however scatterers do account for a decrease in image quality: at impedance boundaries they cause blurring and decreased intensity while within the medium they create speckle. Even though the presence of scatterers in ultrasound must be accepted, their effect on image quality can be managed to some degree by adjusting properties such as transducer frequency; as explained in section 2 a lower frequency will be less subject to the effects of scattering. However, this must be weighed against the many other features that affect image quality.

Shadowing/Enhancement

Almost all ultrasound devices include a swept-gain control function, as described in section 3. Assuming these controls to be properly calibrated, the displayed image corresponding to a given area of the body should be of uniform intensity, or brightness, across all depths. In practice, however, it is almost impossible to perfectly calibrate the swept-gain control; the result is one of two artifacts: shadowing and enhancement. A "shadow" is cast by any imaged tissue whose rate of attenuation of sound is greater than that of the background, surrounding medium. The added loss in intensity as sound propagates through this portion of the medium will mean that attenuation will be greater than the amount that is accounted for by the SGC. As a result, the transmitted sound beam at all points beyond this tissue will be of lower intensity than what is expected, and the image corresponding to those points will be of lower brightness than expected.

The most logical means of accounting for this extraordinary loss of sonic magnitude would be to fine-tune the swept-gain control such that the lost intensity is "added back" to the signal at the proper depth. This would require an advanced knowledge of the region being imaged, would not be very accurate, and would introduce additional noise and other artifacts into the image. Instead, consider the influence of frequency on the degree of shadowing. Like almost every aspect of ultrasound, sound wave frequency has a pronounced effect on shadowing and must be selected carefully to maintain a delicate balance of all dependent factors. Because higher frequency sound waves are subject to a higher rate of attenuation, they are also corrected to a higher degree by the SGC, that is the controls form a "steeper" angle. So when propagating through a high-attenuating material, the degree of shadowing that results after correction also becomes greater. Because the high-attenuating material is of a fixed width, a greater amount of signal loss that is not completely corrected for by the SGC will occur across this width.

The opposite effect of shadowing can occur by the same principle: if a part of the imaged medium has a rate of attenuation that is lower than that of the surrounding medium, there will be less of a loss in intensity than was originally accounted for. As a result all points beyond along the axis of the sound beam will have a higher sound wave intensity and higher projected image brightness level than the baseline, a phenomenon known as enhancement. Like shadowing, enhancement is a function of transducer frequency and must be recognized when analyzing ultrasound images.

Reverberation

The transmitted and reflected sound waves discussed so far have been limited to intended signals that return necessary information. However the tissue medium holds no discrimination for signals that are desired by the ultrasound device and other signals that propagate through; all behave the same way. A significant artifact that can result from unintended sound waves is reverberation. To explain, consider once again a simplified layout containing only the transducer placed on the surface of the skin and a single tissue (say, muscle) held within a surrounding medium (water). The desired effect is for the transmitted sound beam to reflect off of each interface and return to the transducer:

It cannot be ignored that the sound wave will *continue to propagate* and therefore continue to reflect off of each interface, i.e. it will reverberate. Upon returning to the transducer, the sound wave will reflect back at the medium and again undergo its original path. As you can see, this will eventually cause the transducer to receive a signal that corresponds to a location beyond the farthest edge of the tissue layout.

While this incorrect information can be removed by simply limiting the displayed image to a specified depth (either temporally or spatially), similar artifacts can always occur due to reverberation between any two interface. Consider the situation below:

The sound wave will continue to "bounce" between the interfaces at A and B, each time returning part of its signal back to the transducer. Because both interfaces are close to the transducer, the reverberation artifacts appear within the limits of the image, and will continue until the sound wave magnitude is attenuated below a minimum level. There is no real solution to reverberation, other than being aware of its presence and learning to identify situations where it is likely to occur.

Deflection

As described in section 2, refraction occurs whenever an incident sound beam strikes an interface at a non-perpendicular angle. What must also be accounted for is the deflective effect that this has on regeneration of the image. As can be seen below, a transmitted beam that refracts at an interface, strikes a reflecting interface, then refracts back towards the transducer on return will be received and interpreted as being positioned along a straight axis from the transducer. The system can only assume that sound travels in a straight line away from and then back towards the transducer, although when refraction occurs this is not the actual case. The end result is improper positioning of interfaces on the final image.

Resolution

The resolution of an image is perceived as the sharpness or quality of the image; it is a function of the number of pixels in the image, or the size of each of these pixels. A given physiological region can theoretically be imaged at any resolution, depending on the properties of the imaging equipment. Mathematically, resolution is the smallest possible distance between two points on the image such that the two points can still be distinguished from each other. A higher resolution is preferred, this means the viewer can separate two points that are very close to each other; the image contains more information and is visually more detailed. Note that the designation "high resolution" implies "better" resolution, which actually corresponds to resolution having a lower numerical value and smaller pixel size.

The size of a square pixel is of course based on its two dimensions, width and height. In ultrasound terms, the width and height axes correspond to a distance and rotation from the transducer origin, while resolution is expressed in terms of these two lengths. Distance from the transducer is referred to as range while rotation from the main axis is referred to as azimuth; both are usually measured in mm. The resolution in these two dimensions in ultrasound is constrained by properties of the transmitted sound wave that is used and by the setup of the ultrasound machine.

Range resolution is limited by the duration of each transmitted sound pulse. Each pulse propagates away from transducer, along the range axis. Two objects that are close enough to each other relative to the duration of the transmitted pulse will be interpreted as one single, larger object and will be indistinguishable from each other in the final image. Pulse duration is another property that is affected by the transducer frequency setting.

Azimuth resolution is limited by beam width. Two objects whose distance between each other is smaller than the width of the sound beam will similarly be grouped together and imaged as a single object. As previously described, beam width is determined by the physical dimensions of the transducer element and is adjustable to some extent. The narrowest part of the beam, and therefore the highest resolution, occurs in the focal region.

These absolute resolution limits are defined by the sound beam, but in ultrasound practice the more applicable resolution limits are set by the constraints of real-time updating. Recall that the entire displayed ultrasound image must be continuously reacquired and redrawn at a rate fast enough that motion is perceived by the viewer. The human eye updates at 30 fps, so each two-dimensional image must be acquired in 1/30 sec or about 33ms. Since the amount of time available for acquiring an image is limited, resolution ultimately comes down to the speed of sound, which cannot be altered. Given this fixed amount of time to work with during which the sound wave must be transmitted and received at each image line, there is a tradeoff that must be made between the number of imaged lines within the region in question (azimuth resolution) and the depth of each imaged line. First a maximum depth from the transducer that the image must cover is selected; from this value the number of lines that can be scanned within 33ms is calculated and these lines are evenly spaced throughout the imaged region, setting the azimuth resolution.

Resolution describes the degree of image definition not only in the two spatial dimensions but also in the intensity dimension. In a similar manner as with spatial resolution, intensity resolution is quantified by the smallest possible detectable change in intensity between two points. Since the image is stored digitally, the number of possible values that a pixel may have or number of bits of storage at each pixel makes up the image intensity resolution. Intensity resolution can be improved by increasing the magnitude of the transmitted sound wave, allowing smaller fractional changes in received pulses to be detected. Intensity resolution is also limited by the storage space and speed of the ultrasound device that processes all of the information.

The differences between ultrasound and sound in normal hearing range

Characteristic	Sound in normal hearing range	Ultrasound
Frequency	20 Hz – 20 kHz	Over 20 kHz For medical imaging, 1 MHz – 15 MHz
Audibility	Audible to humans	Inaudible to humans
Wavelength	Longer wavelength	Shorter wavelength
Scattering	More easily scattered	Less easily scattered by body tissue

Te piezoelectric effect and the effect of using an alternating potential difference with a piezoelectric crystal

- Certain crystalline materials, with fixed ions in the crystalline lattice, exhibit an effect in which mechanical stress applied to the crystal produces a potential difference between opposite faces. This effect is called the piezoelectric effect.

- Conversely, a potential difference applied to opposite faces of the crystal, say by two electrodes on either side of a flat slab of piezoelectric crystal, causes mechanical deformation of the crystal. If an alternating potential difference is applied, the crystal vibrates, that is, becomes alternately thinner then fatter between the electrodes, at the same the frequency as the applied potential difference.

- If the vibrating crystal is in contact with air, it will produce a sound wave of the same frequency as the alternating potential difference. The frequency of the applied alternating potential difference is chosen to give the desired frequency of ultrasound. Careful sizing of the crystal material, to match its natural resonant vibration to this frequency, makes for the most efficient transfer of electrical energy to ultrasound energy.

- 33 -

Acoustic impedance

- **Acoustic impedance**, Z, is the opposition of a medium to the passage of sound waves. A substance with a high acoustic impedance hinders the movement of sound energy more than a substance with a low acoustic impedance.

- Impedance is proportional to both the density of the medium and the velocity of the sound within it. The units for acoustic impedance can be found by multiplying the units for density by the units for velocity. Hence, acoustic impedance is measured in $kgm^{-2}s^{-1}$.

- The body consists of a range of materials, such as air in the lungs, gas in the bowel, water, blood, muscle, fat and bone. Each body component has a characteristic impedance that depends upon the nature of the matter in it. Gases have very low density, therefore very low acoustic impedance. The impedance of a particular tissue will vary within a range around a typical value.

Substance	Characteristic acoustic impedance
Air	$429\ kgm^{-2}s^{-1}$
Water	$1.43 \times 10^6\ kgm^{-2}s^{-1}$

Sample calculation
The density of blood is $1060\ kgm^{-3}$ and its ultrasound velocity is $1570\ ms^{-1}$
Acoustic impedance, $Z = \rho v = 1060 \times 1570 = 1.59 \times 10^6\ kgm^{-2}s^{-1}$

Ultrasound will move through a medium until it encounters a boundary. When this happens some ultrasound will be reflected from the boundary and some will cross the boundary. The ratio of these two amounts depends upon the difference between their acoustic impedance. A big difference will mean that very little of the sound will cross the boundary. This means that the boundary will give a strong echo. Ultrasound echoes are the basis of examining tissues. Bone has the highest acoustic impedance in the body and so most sound is reflected from the surface of the bone. This means that the sound cannot penetrate the bone. Tissues enclosed by bone, (eg in the skull) hidden by bone or within bone cannot be examined.

For a similar reason air interfaces have almost complete reflection. This means that tissues with enclosed air, such as the lungs, are difficult to image.

On the other hand adjacent tissues with similar acoustic impedances will allow some ultrasound to be transmitted and some reflected. This allows both an echo and further penetration of the ultrasound. Each boundary will give an echo a short time later than the preceding one. This allows us to examine the tissue the sound has just passed through. Thus soft or watery tissues such as muscle, fat and blood can be examined.

The principles of acoustic impedance and reflection and refraction applied to ultrasound

- A short burst (pulse) of ultrasound is produced by a piezoelectric transducer. This pulse will travel through a medium until it reaches the boundary with another medium.
- Some of the pulse will be reflected and will return to the transducer. The distance from the transducer to the boundary (ie the depth of the boundary) can be found by recording the time between the pulse and its echo.
- Some of the pulse will cross the boundary (ie be refracted) into the second medium. This refracted pulse will continue into the second medium until it reaches another boundary, where some of it will be reflected to return to the transducer and some will be refracted a second time. In this way a series of echoes having different time lags from the initial burst will be recorded. Each represents a boundary at a different distance (depth) from the transducer.
- The amount of ultrasound reflected compared to the amount refracted at a boundary will depend upon the different acoustic impedances of each medium. A large difference in impedance means that there is more reflection and less refraction at a boundary.

The **A scan** consists of a series of amplitude peaks on a cathode ray oscilloscope (CRO) trace, each peak corresponding to an echo from a boundary of a certain depth. The CRO trace is actually a time scale but knowing the pulse velocity allows us to determine distance, that is, the depth of the boundary that returned an echo. **A scans** are used in situations where only distance measurements are required. Two such situations are measurements in the eye and foetal skull size. The latter can be used to estimate the developmental stage of the foetus. **A scans** require less complex equipment than other ultrasound techniques.

B scans

- B (brightness) scans show the echo as a brightness signal on the CRO.

- A static **B scan** consists of a series of bright dots.
- Each dot on a static **B scan** corresponds to an echo from a boundary of a certain depth.
- Static **B scans** are not very useful on their own
- **B scans** form the basis of sector and phase scans.

Example of a table

Scan type	Description	Example of use	Reason for use
Phase scan	The ultrasound probe has many transducers. These are arranged to send pulses at slightly different times, that is, with a different phase. In this way the overall wavefront will travel in a certain direction. This allows the pulse to be directed in a sweep to build up a cross sectional image.	obstetrics abdominal investigations cardiography	shows a two dimensional image produces good image quality
Sector scan	Successive B scans are made as the transducer probe is rocked sideways on the patient. Each static B scan is added to form a fan-shaped (sector) brightness image. This is a cross-sectional image.	imaging of the infant brain through the fontanel	shows a two dimensional image only needs a small entry 'window'.

the Doppler effect in sound waves and how it is used in ultrasonics to obtain flow characteristics of blood moving through the heart

- The **Doppler effect** is the apparent change in wavelength of a wave when it is produced by a source moving relative to a stationary observer. When a source of sound waves moves towards an observer, the waves are 'bunched up'; their wavelength is shorter and the frequency heard by the observer is higher. The converse is true when the source is moving away from the observer. The Doppler effect also happens if the source is stationary and the observer is moving.

- 36 -

- If a pulse of ultrasound reflects off a stationary boundary it will return with the same frequency and wavelength as was emitted. If the boundary is moving away from the transducer there will be a Doppler shift effect. The waves will undergo a Doppler shift on their outward and reflected journeys, producing a double Doppler shift.

- Ultrasound used in blood flow measurement is typically in the range 5 to 15 MHz. The 'moving boundary' comprises the surfaces of multiple red blood cells, as an individual red blood cell is too small to be a boundary on its own. The Doppler shift is typically a change in frequency of up to 3 kHz. This value is positive when blood flows towards the probe, and negative when the blood flows away.

- Sophisticated computer software can assign colours to an ultrasound scan on the basis of its Doppler shift. In this way flow velocity can be seen. A colour change can indicate increased velocity, indicating a narrowed artery. Colour intensity can indicate flow volume. Mixed colours can indicate flow turbulence due to a partial blockage. The wrong colour can indicate a leaking heart valve. Doppler shifts can be in the audible range and so can be heard. An experienced operator can make a diagnosis using this sound.

The ratio of reflected to initial intensity as: $$\frac{I_r}{I_o} = \frac{[Z_2 - Z_1]^2}{[Z_2 + Z_1]^2}$$

- You should be able to clearly indicate that 'intensity' is a measure of the energy in the pulse of ultrasound and that it depends upon the amplitude of the waves in a pulse of a certain frequency. You should also be able to indicate that acoustic impedance is a function of the density of a material and the velocity of the waves in that material.

Resolution, Beamforming and the Point Spread Function

A typical transducer uses an array of piezoelectric elements to transmit a sound pulse into the body and to receive the echoes that return from scattering structures within. This array is often referred to as the imaging system's **aperture**. The transmit signals passing to, and the received signals passing from the array elements can be individually delayed in time, hence the term **phased array**. This is done to electronically steer and focus each of a sequence of acoustic pulses through the plane or volume to be imaged in the body. This produces a 2- or 3-D map of the scattered echoes, or **tissue echogenicity** that is presented to the clinician for interpretation. The process of steering and focusing these acoustic pulses is known as **beamforming**. This process is shown schematically in Figure 1.1.

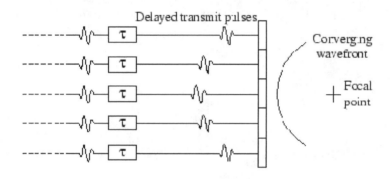

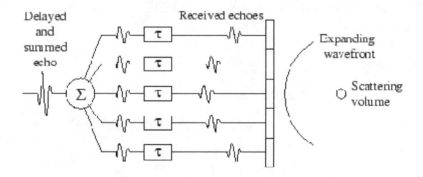

Figure 1.1: A conceptual diagram of phased array beamforming. (Top) Appropriately delayed pulses are transmitted from an array of piezoelectric elements to achieve steering and focusing at the point of interest. (For simplicity, only focusing delays are shown here.) (Bottom) The echoes returning are likewise delayed before they are summed together to form a strong echo signal from the region of interest.

The ability of a particular ultrasound system to discriminate closely spaced scatterers is specified by its spatial resolution, which is typically defined as the minimum scatterer spacing at which this discrimination is possible. The system resolution has three components in Cartesian space, reflecting the spatial extent of the ultrasound pulse at the focus. The coordinates of this space are in the axial, lateral, and elevation dimensions. The axial, or **range**, dimension indicates the predominant direction of sound propagation, extending from the transducer into the body. The axial and the lateral dimension together define the tomographic plane, or slice, of the displayed image. These dimensions relative to the face of a linear array transducer are shown in Figure 1.2. The elevation dimension contains the slice thickness.

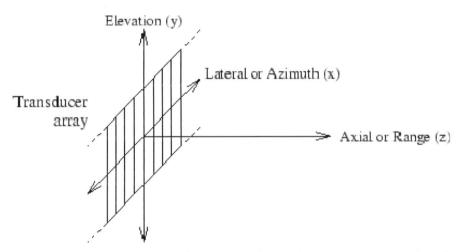

Figure 1.2: A diagram of the spatial coordinate system used to describe the field and resolution of an ultrasound transducer array. Here the transducer is a 1-D array, subdivided into elements in the lateral dimension. The transmitted sound pulse travels out in the axial dimension.

A modern ultrasound scanner operating in brightness mode, or **B-mode**, presents the viewer with a gray-scale image that represents a map of echo amplitude, or **brightness,** as a function of position in the region being scanned. In B-mode the ultrasound system interrogates the region of interest with wide bandwidth sound pulses. Such a pulse from a typical array is shown in Figure 1.3.

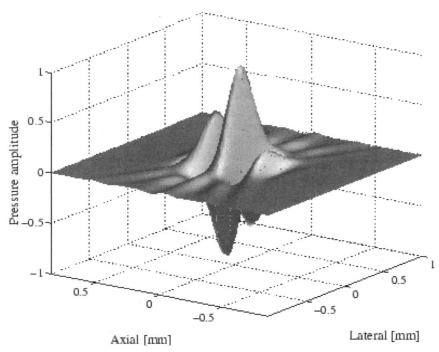

Figure 1.3: The acoustic pulse from a typical array (7.5 MHz, 60% bandwidth, 128 elements of width equal to the wavelength), shown at the acoustic focus. The pulse is displayed as a map of pressure amplitude and is traveling in the positive direction along axial dimension.

The acoustic pulse in Figure 1.3 is shown as a function of acoustic pressure over the lateral and axial dimensions. In fact the pulse is a three-dimensional function, with extent in elevation as well. In the terminology of linear systems theory it is the impulse response of the system, and the response of the ultrasound system at the focus is fully characterized by this function. As it represents the output of the ultrasound system during interrogation of an ideal point target, it is also known as the system's **point spread function** (PSF). The character of the PSF in the axial dimension is determined predominantly by the center frequency and bandwidth of the acoustic signal generated at each transducer element, while its character in the lateral and elevation dimensions is determined predominantly by the aperture and element geometries and the beamforming applied. The term PSF is often used to refer to two-dimensional representations of the system response in pressure amplitude versus space, such as that shown in Figure 1.3, with the implicit understanding that the actual response has three-dimensional extent.

In analyzing hypothetical ultrasound systems, predicting the form of the PSF is critical. However, the analytic solution for the PSF for an arbitrary array geometry is usually intractable. Throughout this document, an acoustic field simulation program developed by Jensen and Svendsen was used to predict the acoustic field under the various conditions and array geometries of interest. This program is based on a method developed by Tupholme and Stephanishen. It calculates the convolution of a transmit excitation function, such as a sine wave with Gaussian envelope, with the spatial impulse response of the transducer. The spatial impulse response is the hypothetical pressure pattern created upon excitation of the array with a perfect impulse. The spatial impulse response is not a physically realizable, but serves as a useful calculation tool in this context. This method can accommodate arbitrary geometries by division of the aperture into smaller, rectangular elements. The spatial impulse response for each element is calculated separately, and then these solutions are combined by superposition to produce that for the entire aperture.

The **sound** in ultrasound is a physical longitudinal wave. The compression and rarefaction of the medium at the wavefront causes particle translations on the order of microns. The tissue at the cellular level is perturbed on a bulk level, i.e. the wavelength is much greater than the size of cells.

Here are some numbers of interest to put ultrasound in perspective. At 1 MHz, 100 mW/cm^2 (FDA upper acoustic power limit):

Wavelengthmm

Phase velocity 1540 m/s = 1.54 mm/μs

Peak particle displacement 0.0057 μm

Peak particle velocity 3.8 cm/sec

Peak particle acceleration 22,452 g

Peak pressure 1.8 atm

Radiation force 0.007 g/cm^2

Heat equivalent 0.024 cal/sec cm^2 (total absorption)

The Scattering and Reflection of Sound

Medical ultrasound imaging relies utterly on the fact that biological tissues scatter or reflect incident sound. Although the phenomenon are closely related, in this text scattering refers to the interaction between sound waves and particles that are much smaller than the sound's wavelength λ, while reflection refers to such interaction with particles or objects larger than λ.

The scattering or reflection of acoustic waves arise from inhomogeneities in the medium's density and/or compressibility. Sound is primarily scattered or reflected by a discontinuity in the medium's mechanical properties, to a degree proportional to the discontinuity. (By contrast, continuous changes in a medium's material properties cause the direction of propagation to change gradually.) The elasticity and density of a material are related to its sound speed, and thus sound is scattered or reflected most strongly by significant discontinuities in the density and/or sound speed of the medium.

Rayleigh – Tyndall scattering

Backscattering of ultrasound from blood. The echoes detected from blood (e.g. in Doppler ultrasound) are created through interference between scattered wavelets from numerous point scatterers. The intensity of the backscattered echoes is proportional to the total number of scatterers, which means that the echo amplitude is proportional to the square root of the total number of scatterers. At normal blood flow, the number of point scatterers in blood is proportional to the number of red blood cells (i.e. the amount of blood). When blood flow is turbulent, or accelerating fast (e.g. in a stenosis), the number of inhomogeneities in the red blood cell concentration will increase, thus giving rise to stronger echoes than can be accounted for by merely the amount of blood. The intensity of the backscattered ultrasound is also proportional to the fourth power of ultrasound frequency. Doubling the ultrasonic frequency makes the echoes from blood 16 times as strong. (On the other hand, higher frequency ultrasound suffers from higher attenuation in the tissues.)

Ultrasonic Absorption

loss of ultrasound energy by conversion into heat. Absorption is proportional to the ultrasound frequency; the higher the frequency, the greater the loss of energy as heat.

Focusing

In ultrasound imaging, the focusing of the ultrasound beam by means of acoustic lenses or electronic focusing. The ultrasound transmitted from the transducer crystal can be considered to be composed of multiple wavelets that interact constructively to create a wavefront (see Huygens principle). In an acoustic lens, the speed of sound is higher than in the soft tissues in front of the lens, and wavelets that have traveled the longest distance through a concave lens, i.e. the more peripheral ones, will be ahead of the more centrally located wavelets after the lens is passed. The wavefront is therefore curved, and the ultrasound beam becomes focused. A concave transducer surface would give the same effect. The principle is valid for electronic focusing as well.

Ultrasound beam

The confined, directional beam of ultrasound travelling as a longitudinal wave from the transducer face into the propagation medium. Two separate regions along the beam can be identified, the near field or Fresnel zone, and the far field or Fraunhofer zone. A confined, slightly converging beam shape is maintained in the near field owing to constructive and destructive interference patterns of individual sound wavelets emitted from the surface of the transducer crystal. The length of the near field is equal to $r^2/\lambda = d^2/4\,\lambda$, where r is the radius and d the diameter of the transducer crystal, and λ is the ultrasound wavelength in the medium of propagation. Maximum ultrasound intensity occurs at the near field - far field interface. Beam divergence in the far field results in a continuous loss of ultrasound intensity with distance from the transducer. The angle of divergence in the far field, q, is approximately equal to arcsin(1.22 λ/d) (or sin q = 1.22l λ/d). Note that with increasing transducer frequency (decreasing wavelength), the length of the near field increases and the angle of divergence in the far field decreases. Both changes improve lateral resolution in deep structures, but this beneficial effect of high transducer frequency is counteracted by the decrease in penetration. An increase in the diameter of the transducer crystal will also increase the length of the near field and decrease the angle of divergence, but with the drawback of a wider ultrasound beam and therefore decreased lateral resolution in the near field.

Intensity of sound

Acoustic energy (joule) per unit time (second) and unit area (square metre). Acoustic power is acoustic energy per unit time and is measured in watts (W), 1 W being 1 joule/s. The intensity of sound is thus the acoustic power per unit area, measured in W/m^2. The intensity is determined by the amplitudes or excursions of the particles conducting the waves; the larger the amplitudes of oscillation, the higher the intensity. The actual relationship is $I = p^2/2Z$, where I is intensity, p is pressure amplitude, and Z is acoustic impedance.

Speed of sound

The propagation speed of a sound wave (e.g. ultrasound) through a medium. The propagation speed is determined by the physical properties of the medium, and is independent of the (ultra)sound frequency. The major parameters affecting the speed of sound (c) are the elasticity (K) and density (ρ) of the medium, their relationship being $c = \surd(K/\rho)$.

High elasticity implies large elastic forces between the particles of the medium and a high resistance against compression (low compressibility). Speed increases with decreasing compressibility (increasing elasticity) because less compressible media have more densely packed molecules which need to move only a small distance before their motion is transmitted to the neighboring molecules. Speed decreases with increasing density because dense materials tend to have large, heavy molecules that are difficult to start and stop in the rhythmic motion involved in the propagation of sound. Tissues may be considered liquids, and in liquids, compressibility and density are generally inversely proportional. The speed of sound is therefore very similar in all tissues, the average speed in human soft tissue being approximately 1540 m/s.

Longitudinal wave

A waveform transmitted through a medium where the particles of the medium oscillate in the direction of the wave propagation. Sound propagates as longitudinal waves. A longitudinal wave is produced when a vibrator, e.g. a piezoelectric crystal in an ultrasound transducer, transmits its back and forth oscillation into a continuous, elastic medium. The particles of the medium are made to oscillate in the direction of the wave propagation, but are otherwise stationary. The wave propagates as bands of compression and rarefaction. One wavelength is the distance between two bands of compression, or rarefaction. Maximum compression corresponds to maximum pressure.

Pulse repetition frequency (PRF)

In pulsed ultrasound, the number of pulses transmitted per second. For imaging, the PRF is usually in the range of 1 000 to 5 000 pulses per second, i.e. 15 kHz. The PRF is limited by the range to be examined. To avoid range ambiguity, the echoes from the deepest structures must be allowed to return to the transducer before the next pulse is transmitted. In pulsed Doppler ultrasound, the PRF determines the maximum measurable velocity.

Ultrasound pulse

A short-duration wave of ultrasound. Pulses of ultrasound, as opposed to continuous wave ultrasound, are used in all ultrasound applications based on the pulse - echo method, such as A-mode, M-mode, B-mode, colour Doppler sonography, power Doppler sonography, and pulsed Doppler ultrasound. The pulse duration and spatial pulse length are determined by factors such as the Q factor of the transducer crystal and by the characteristics of the backing block of the transducer. Typically, B-mode applications use very short pulses to ensure high axial resolution, while Doppler ultrasound requires longer lasting pulses to provide a more narrow spectrum of ultrasound frequencies. There is a reciprocal relationship between the pulse duration and the pulse bandwidth (defined as width of energy spectrum at half height): pulse bandwidth (MHz) ~1/pulse duration (ms).

A-mode

Amplitude mode, a one-dimensional ultrasonic display showing echoes along the ultrasonic beam as vertical spikes on a horizontal time axis indicating the depth of the reflectors. The amplitudes of the spikes reflect the echo strengths after time gain compensation TGC , and the left-right position of the spikes is determined by the time lag between transmission of the ultrasonic pulse and arrival of the echo at the transducer. The later the arrival of the echoes, the further to the right their display.

B-mode

Brightness mode, a two-dimensional ultrasound image display composed of bright dots representing the ultrasound echoes. The brightness of each dot is determined by the echo amplitude (after time gain compensation TGC). A B-mode image is produced by sweeping a narrow ultrasound beam through the region of interest while transmitting pulses and detecting echoes along a series of closely spaced scan lines. The scanning may be performed with a single transducer mounted on an articulating arm that provides information on the ultrasound beam direction (compound B scan, static B scanner), or with a real-time scanner such as a mechanical scanner or an electronic array scanner. A linear array transducer with multiple crystal elements is used. At each scan line position, one ultrasound pulse is transmitted and all echoes from the surface to the deepest range are recorded before the ultrasound beam moves on to the next scan line position where pulse transmission and echo recording are repeated. In the B-mode image, the vertical (depth) position of each bright dot is determined by the time delay from pulse transmission to return of the echo, and the horizontal position by the location of the receiving transducer element. A shadowing artefact (distal to the bone and to the lateral edges of the fluid-filled cyst), and an enhancement artefact (distal to the cyst) are also shown.

M-mode

Motion mode, also called time motion (TM) mode. An ultrasonic display showing A-mode data (echoes) as dots along a vertical depth axis, as opposed to the normal A-mode presentation of spikes along a horizontal depth (time) axis. The brightness of the dots is determined by the echo strength. For each pulse repetition period (PRP), a new set of vertical A-mode data is acquired and the old A-mode data are pushed to the left on the monitor to make room for the new data that are appearing on the right side of the screen. In this way, the dots are made to scroll across the screen (or alternatively on a strip of paper), thus creating bright curves indicating vertical positional changes of the reflectors with time. The M-mode curves provide very detailed information on the motional behavior of reflecting structures along the ultrasound beam and the method is especially popular in cardiology to show the motion patterns of the various cardiac valve leaflets.

The Q factor of an ultrasound transducer is defined as:

$$Q = f0 / (f2 - f1)$$

where f0 is the resonant frequency (centre frequency) of the transducer crystal, f2 is the frequency above resonance at which the intensity is reduced by half, and f1 is the frequency below resonance at which the intensity is reduced by half. f2 - f1 is thus an expression of the band width of the sound.

The Q factor refers to two characteristics of the transducer: the "purity" (bandwidth) of the sound and the persistence of the sound (the ring down time). Bandwidth and sound duration are related. Theoretically, only infinite sine waves have a single frequency. The beginning and end of an ultrasound pulse introduce a range of frequencies; the shorter the pulse, the wider its frequency spectrum. A "high Q" transducer will respond to a short voltage pulse with a relatively long lasting vibration, emitting ultrasound with a narrow bandwidth (nearly "pure" sound). A "low Q" transducer, on the other hand, will vibrate for only a short time period, emitting a short pulse of ultrasound consisting of a broad range of frequencies. Adding a backing block to an ultrasound transducer reduces the Q factor by shortening the ringdown time and consequently the pulse duration, which increases the bandwidth of the ultrasound pulse. "Low Q" transducers are preferable in ultrasound imaging systems where a small spatial pulse length is needed for high axial resolution. Doppler ultrasound applications require transducers with higher Q factor to produce narrow bandwidth ultrasound which is needed for detection of the frequency changes caused by blood flow.

Spatial pulse length

The length of the ultrasound pulse in pulsed ultrasound applications. The spatial pulse length is equal to the number of waves (cycles) in the pulse multiplied by their wavelength. The pulse length is determined by the Q factor of the transducer crystal and by the characteristics of the backing block of the transducer. The spatial pulse length determines the axial resolution of the pulsed ultrasound system.

Axial resolution

The spatial resolution of ultrasound in the ultrasound beam direction, also known as the depth, linear, longitudinal and range resolution. The axial resolution is the minimum distance in the beam direction between two reflectors which can be identified as separate echoes. The axial resolution is slightly more than half the spatial pulse length, which is the number of waves in the transmitted ultrasound pulse (determined by the Q factor) multiplied by their wavelength (determined by the transducer frequency).

Artefact in ultrasound

display of incorrect anatomy or velocity in ultrasound applications. In B mode imaging, artefacts may appear whenever there is a violation of the following assumptions:

1.	The ultrasound beam is narrow with uniform width.
2.	The speed of sound is 1540 m/s in soft tissues.
3.	The attenuation of ultrasound is uniform.
4.	The ultrasound travels in a straight line directly to the reflecting object and back to the transducer.
5.	Echoes from all depths are allowed to reach the transducer before the next ultrasound pulse is emitted.

Assumption 1) may be violated by a wide beam, which causes image smearing of echogenic objects that are smaller than the beam diameter (beam width artefact), or by side lobes or grating lobes (side lobe artefact). Assumption 2) that the speed of sound is constant at 1 540 m/s, is true for most soft tissues, but it is lower in fat (1 450 m/s) and especially in silicone implants (600 m/s). This causes errors in range and distance, and may cause the so-called speed artefact. Variations in attenuation (assumption 3) may cause artificially increased image brightness (enhancement artefact) or decreased image brightness (shadowing artefact). Several artefacts are caused by violation of assumption 4, such as the mirror image artefact or multipath reflection artefact, the reverberation artefact (also named ring-down artefact or comet tail artefact), and split image artefact. Assumption 5 may be violated by a too high pulse repetition frequency PRF, giving rise to the ambiguity artefact.

In Doppler ultrasound applications, artefacts appear whenever the Doppler frequency shift exceeds the Nyquist limit. This causes aliasing, which may be seen as frequency fold over or frequency wrap around in spectral Doppler, or as a mosaic effect in colour Doppler sonography. Use of gas microbubble contrast media may cause bubble noise and blooming artefact.

Shadowing artefact

In ultrasound imaging, a hypoechoic (dark) area distal to an object. The low signal is caused by attenuation (absorption, reflection or refraction) of the ultrasound beam. Shadowing artefacts are typically seen as dark streaking behind highly attenuating objects such as bones and calculi (in e.g. gall bladder or kidney). Dark streaks are also seen distal to the lateral borders of fluid-containing structures (e.g. gall bladder, cysts) due to reflection and refraction of the ultrasound beam from the curved surface.

Ambiguity artefact

Ultrasound image artefact occurring when the pulse repetition frequency PRF is too high to allow the deepest echoes to return to the transducer before the next ultrasound pulse is transmitted. The deepest echoes arrive at the transducer shortly after the next pulse transmission and are consequently mismapped to shallow positions in the image.

Blooming artefact

Smearing of colour signals outside a vessel in colour Doppler sonography, caused by gas microbubble contrast medium. The phenomenon may be due to multiple reflections of the ultrasound back and forth between the bubbles, similar to the reverberation artefact of B mode imaging, and perhaps also to high amplitude echoes caused by collapse of the microbubbles in the ultrasound beam.

Key Points

Absorption is the transfer of energy from the ultrasound beam to the tissue. It is proportional to frequency.

Apodization is a method for reducing side lobes in some arrays. It gradually decreases the vibration of the transducer surface with distance from its center. It is usually accomplished by using more power to excite the innermost elements.

Axial resolution is the minimum separation between two interfaces located in a direction parallel to the beam so that they can be imaged as two different interfaces.

Decibel is a way to express the ratio of two sound intensities: $dB = 10\log_{10}I1/I2$ being I1 the reference. For instance: +3 dB = I multiplied by 2 and -3 db = I divided by 2

Diffraction is the change in the directions and intensities of a group of waves after passing by an obstacle or through an aperture.

Duty factor is the lapse of time the transducer is actively transmitting sound.

Echo ranging is the relationship between transit time and reflector depth expressed as t = 2d/c.

Grating lobes as side lobes are secondary ultrasound beams projecting off-axis at predictable angles to the main beam. Side lobes are too small to produce important artifacts.

Half Value Layer (HVL) is the distance the sound beam penetrates into a tissue when its intensity has been reduced to one half of its initial value.

Huygens' principle states that an expanding sphere of waves behaves as if each point on the wave front were a new source of radiation of the same frequency and phase.

Impedance is the product of the density of a material and the speed of sound in that material.

Pulse average intensity I(PA) is the average intensity during the pulse.

Lateral resolution is the minimum separation of two interfaces aligned along a direction perpendicular to the ultrasound beam. It depends on the beam width.

Partial Volume Artifact (slice thickness or volume averaging artifact), that occurs when the slice thickness is wider than the scanned structure.

Q-value means the degree that a transducer is finely tuned to specific narrow frequency range. For instance: Low Q means wide bandwitdh and High Q means narrow bandwidth.

Range resolution is the ability to determine the depth of reflectors.

Rayleigh scatterers are objects whose dimensions are much less than the ultrasound wavelength. Scattering increases with frequency raised to the 4th power and provides much of the diagnostic information from ultrasound.

Refraction is the bending of a wave beam when it crosses at an oblique angle the interface of two materials, through which the waves propagate at different velocities

Snell's law governs the direction of the transmitted beam when refraction occurs: $\sin q_t = (c_2/c_1) \times \sin q_i$ (q_t and q_i are transmit and incident angles respectively)

Spatial Average Intensity (SA) is the acoustic power within the beam, divided by the beam area.

Spatial Peak Intensity (SP) is the point in the sound field with maximum intensity.

Side lobes are energy in the sound beam falling outside the main beam.

Spatial resolution means how closely two reflectors -or scattering regions, can be to one another while they can be identified as different reflectors.

Subdicing is a technique used to overcome grating lobes: each major transducer element is divided into smaller parts, each one being a half wave length.

Temporal (instantaneous) Peak Intensity I(TP) or I(IP) is the maximum intensity during the pulse.

Time Average Intensity I(TA): average intensity calculated over the time between pulses:
ITA= I(PA) x Duty factor.

Wavelength is l=c/f (c = propagation speed; f = frequency)

Ultrasound Physics

Ultrasound, unlike light and x-rays, needs a medium for travel. For our purposes, this propagating medium is tissue or fluid. Ultrasound cannot travel though air, even the smallest amount. Air is therefore an acoustic barrier while the presence of fluid is quite helpful for sonograms. This is exactly the opposite of radiology, where air is "our friend", yielding contrast, while fluid is "our enemy" obscuring organs from view. Diagnostic ultrasound utilizes sound waves at a very high frequency, in the range of 2-10 megahertz (MHz). This is in contrast to audible sound which is in the 20-20,000 Hz range.

Diagnostic ultrasound utilizes the "pulse echo" principle to create a visible image of tissue and tissue interfaces within the body. An electrical impulse is applied to a piezoelectric (pressure electric) crystal or crystals within the transducer (probe). These crystals convert electrical energy into mechanical energy (ultrasound). The ultrasound travels within the soft tissues of the body at an average of 1540 m/sec. As the sound reaches each organ or tissue, a portion of the sound is reflected (echoes) back to the transducer, which now converts the mechanical energy (returning ultrasound) into electrical energy. This electrical information is then processed by the computer within the ultrasound machine, forming an image on the display screen. The image on the screen is created by a multitude of "dots", each dot located at the appropriate depth of the reflected echo, determined by how long it took for that particular echo to return to the transducer. The brightness or whiteness of each dot is determined by the strength of the returning echo. No returning echoes from a particular location are depicted as black dots (anechoic). The pulses of sound emitted by the transducer occur only 0.1% of the time, allowing the transducer to listen for returning echoes 99.9% of the time. This is an important concept, as the biological effects of ultrasound (heat deposition in tissue) have proven to be negligible since very little time is spent transmitting the ultrasound beam. This is in contrast to therapeutic ultrasound, which utilizes continuous transmission of ultrasound.

As ultrasound travels through tissue, it grows weaker (diminished volume), known as attenuation. Attenuation occurs by three processes. Absorption occurs when the energy is captured by the tissue and converted to heat. Scattering occurs when the ultrasound beam encounters irregular interfaces, sending it in all directions (thus only a small percentage of it returns to the transducer to contribute to image formation). Reflection of sound is the third process in attenuation of the ultrasound beam, occurring at interfaces between tissues of different acoustic properties. The net effect is attenuation of approximately 0.5 dB/cm/MHZ. Higher frequency ultrasound is attenuated more rapidly over distance traveled than lower frequencies. Therefore, lower frequency transducers (e.g., 2.5 MHz) are used to image deeper structures. Higher frequency transducers (e.g., 7.5 MHz) offer much better resolution at the expense of less depth penetration.

Terminology

Ultrasound terminology describes organs or structures as to how echogenic they are relative to other tissues in the same patient. The following are those most commonly used:

Hypoechoic-less intense echo production (object appears darker gray)

Hyperechoic-more intense or more highly reflective (object appears lighter gray to white)

Anechoic-absence of echoes (objects appear black)

Isoechoic-of the dame echogenicity

Mixed echogenicity-having a complex echo pattern of tow or more echogenicities

The relative echogenicities of normal abdominal organs from least echogenic (darkest) to most echogenic (brightest, whitest) are:

renal medulla<renal cortex<liver,<spleen<prostate gland

Spatial resolution is the ability to identify two closely spaced objects. The smaller the distance that can be separated, the better the resolution. Axial resolution is the ability to resolve closely spaced objects along the axis of the ultrasound beam. Lateral resolution is the ability to resolve closely spaced objects perpendicular to the ultrasound beam's axis (side-by-side). Axial resolution is greater than lateral resolution.

Artifacts

Distant Enhancement - an artifact that occurs deep to fluid-filled structures (e.g., gallbladder), resulting in brighter echoes because the ultrasound is not attenuated by the fluid.

Acoustic Shadowing - failure of the ultrasound beam to pass through an object because of reflection and/or absorption of the ultrasound. The result is an anechoic (black) zone beyond the surface of the reflector. This occurs with mineral or gas (e.g., bone, cystic calculus, lung.)

Reverberation - an artifact that is the result of sound bouncing back and forth between two interfaces, resulting in repeated time delays and the display of parallel lines at regular intervals deep to the actual returning echo. This is the common artifact seen when imaging aerated lung or gas within a loop of intestine or stomach. Ring-down artifacts, occurring at the skin-transducer surface and comet-tail artifacts, which occur with metal or air interfaces are other common examples of reverberation artifact.

Refraction - a bending or change in direction of the ultrasound beam as it encounters a rounded structure resulting in an area of echo drop-out, mimicking an acoustic shadow. This commonly occurs along the edge of the kidney, or from within the kidney at the corticomedullary junction.

Mirror-image - artifactual image appearing on the opposite side of a strong, curved reflector, the result of multiple internal reverberations between the object and the reflector, creating a time delay in the return of these internal echoes to the transducer. Thus an erroneously placed structure in addition to the "real" structure is displayed on the video screen. The common mirror-image artifact is the liver and gallbladder, seen on the "other side" of the diaphragm. This could be mistaken for a diaphragmatic hernia.

Four types of Doppler Ultrasound

Continuous Wave (CW)

This mode requires a transducer with separate elements for transmitting and receiving. Because of the continuous wave of ultrasound, a single transducer element cannot alternate between transmitting and receiving. CW ultrasound does not have the ability to discriminate depth of velocities. It samples velocities all along its path. Its primary use is to accurately measure high blood flows, such as across a stenotic valve, which pulse wave and color Doppler are unable to do.

Pulse Wave (PW)

The principal advantage of a PW Doppler is that blood flow velocity can be determined at a specific site. Limitations are that it is cannot measure high velocities (due to the Nyquist limit, called aliasing).

CW and PW Doppler are displayed on a x-y axis, known as spectral Doppler. Each vertical line in the display represents a specific instant in time. The length represents the range of velocities present. The top of the line indicates the maximum velocity. Sound can be used to listen to blood flow as well.

Color
Color Doppler is form of PW Doppler and thus subject to the same limitations of high velocity. The display color is determined by the direction and relative flow velocity. Typically the color display is superimposed on a conventional B-mode. In a typical color Doppler display, red indicates flow toward the transducer and blue indicates flow in the opposite direction. Other colors represent turbulence or aliasing artifact.

Energy or Power Doppler

This is the newest form of Doppler. It is capable of detecting the smallest of blood flow. However, there is no display of velocity or direction. It allows the visualization of smaller vessels. It contains only one color scale and produces a homogeneous color appearance overlying a B-mode image. Power Doppler is only available on sophisticated and very expensive equipment.

Piezoelectric Effect

The phenomenon that certain crystals change their physical dimensions when subjected to an electric field, and vice versa; when deformed by external pressure, an electric field is created across the crystal (from the Greek word piezein = pressure). Piezoelectric crystals are used in ultrasound transducers to transmit and receive ultrasound.

Effect of applied electric field

The piezoelectric crystal in ultrasound transducers has electrodes attached to its front and back for the application and detection of electrical charges. The crystal consists of numerous dipoles, and in the normal state, the individual dipoles have an oblique orientation with no net surface charge. An electric field applied across the crystal will realign the dipoles due to repulsive or attractive electric forces resulting in compression or expansion of the crystal, depending on the direction of the electric field. (For transmission of a short ultrasound pulse, a voltage spike of very short duration is applied, causing the crystal to initially contract and then vibrate for a short time with its resonant frequency.)

Effect of external pressure

When echoes are received, the longitudinal ultrasound waves will compress and expand the crystal. This deformation realigns the dipoles, creating net charges on the crystal surface. In practice, the compression and expansion only amount to a few microns.

Sensitivity in Ultrasound

Why is high sensitivity important?

Higher sensitivity (larger d_1 or g_1 constant) represents a larger response and improved signal-to-noise ratio for a given stimulus. Selecting the proper piezoelectric material for a given application often involves a trade-off between sensitivity and other properties such as Curie point or Dielectric constant. For example, materials with the highest charge constant (d_1) have lower Curie points than materials with lower charge constants.

Why is high sensitivity needed in medical ultrasound?

The piezoelectric material both projects and senses the acoustic wave. High sensitivity is necessary to maximize the signal-to-noise ratio for the returned acoustic wave.

Piezoelectricity

In 1880, Jacques and Pierre Curie discovered an unusual characteristic of certain crystalline minerals: when subjected to a mechanical force, the crystals became electrically polarized. Tension and compression generated voltages of opposite polarity, and in proportion to the applied force. Subsequently, the converse of this relationship was confirmed: if one of these voltage-generating crystals was exposed to an electric field it lengthened or shortened according to the polarity of the field, and in proportion to the strength of the field. These behaviors were labeled the piezoelectric effect and the inverse piezoelectric effect, respectively, from the Greek word piezein, meaning to press or squeeze.

Although the magnitudes of piezoelectric voltages, movements, or forces are small, and often require amplification (a typical disc of piezoelectric ceramic will increase or decrease in thickness by only a small fraction of a millimeter, for example) piezoelectric materials have been adapted to an impressive range of applications. The piezoelectric effect is used in sensing applications, such as in force or displacement sensors. The inverse piezoelectric effect is used in actuation applications, such as in motors and devices that precisely control positioning, and in generating sonic and ultrasonic signals.

In the 20th century metal oxide-based piezoelectric ceramics and other man-made materials enabled designers to employ the piezoelectric effect and the inverse piezoelectric effect in many new applications. These materials generally are physically strong and chemically inert, and they are relatively inexpensive to manufacture. The composition, shape, and dimensions of a piezoelectric ceramic element can be tailored to meet the requirements of a specific purpose. Ceramics manufactured from formulations of lead zirconate / lead titanate exhibit greater sensitivity and higher operating temperatures, relative to ceramics of other compositions, and "PZT" materials currently are the most widely used piezoelectric ceramics.

How are piezoelectric ceramics made?

A traditional piezoelectric ceramic is a mass of perovskite crystals, each consisting of a small, tetravalent metal ion, usually titanium or zirconium, in a lattice of larger, divalent metal ions, usually lead or barium, and O_2- ions. Under conditions that confer tetragonal or rhombohedral symmetry on the crystals, each crystal has a dipole moment.

To prepare a piezoelectric ceramic, fine powders of the component metal oxides are mixed in specific proportions, then heated to form a uniform powder. The powder is mixed with an organic binder and is formed into structural elements having the desired shape (discs, rods, plates, etc.). The elements are fired according to a specific time and temperature program, during which the powder particles sinter and the material attains a dense crystalline structure. The elements are cooled, then shaped or trimmed to specifications, and electrodes are applied to the appropriate surfaces.

Above a critical temperature, the *Curie point*, each perovskite crystal in the fired ceramic element exhibits a simple cubic symmetry with no dipole moment. At temperatures below the Curie point, however, each crystal has tetragonal or rhombohedral symmetry and a dipole moment. Adjoining dipoles form regions of local alignment called *domains*. The alignment gives a net dipole moment to the domain, and thus a net polarization. The direction of polarization among neighboring domains is random, however, so the ceramic element has no overall polarization.

The domains in a ceramic element are aligned by exposing the element to a strong, direct current electric field, usually at a temperature slightly below the Curie point. Through this polarizing *(poling)* treatment, domains most nearly aligned with the electric field expand at the expense of domains that are not aligned with the field, and the element lengthens in the direction of the field. When the electric field is removed most of the dipoles are locked into a configuration of near alignment. The element now has a permanent polarization, the remanent polarization, and is permanently elongated.

What can piezoelectric ceramics do?
Mechanical compression or tension on a poled piezoelectric ceramic element changes the dipole moment, creating a voltage. Compression along the direction of polarization, or tension perpendicular to the direction of polarization, generates voltage of the same polarity as the poling voltage. Tension along the direction of polarization, or compression perpendicular to the direction of polarization, generates a voltage with polarity opposite that of the poling voltage. These actions are generator actions -- the ceramic element converts the mechanical energy of compression or tension into electrical energy. This behavior is used in fuel-igniting devices, solid state batteries, force-sensing devices, and other products. Values for compressive stress and the voltage (or field strength) generated by applying stress to a piezoelectric ceramic element are linearly proportional up to a material-specific stress. The same is true for applied voltage and generated strain.

If a voltage of the same polarity as the poling voltage is applied to a ceramic element, in the direction of the poling voltage, the element will lengthen and its diameter will become smaller. If a voltage of polarity opposite that of the poling voltage is applied, the element will become shorter and broader. If an alternating voltage is applied, the element will lengthen and shorten cyclically, at the frequency of the applied voltage. This is motor action -- electrical energy is converted into mechanical energy. The principle is adapted to piezoelectric motors, sound or ultrasound generating devices, and many other products.

Properties of Acoustic Plane Wave

Wavelength, Frequency and Velocity

Among the properties of waves propagating in isotropic solid materials are wavelength, frequency, and velocity. The wavelength is directly proportional to the velocity of the wave and inversely proportional to the frequency of the wave. This relationship is shown by the following equation.

$$Wavelength(\lambda) = \frac{Velocity(v)}{Frequency(f)}$$

Refraction and Snell's Law

When an ultrasound wave passes through an interface between two materials at an oblique angle, and the materials have different indices of refraction, it produces both reflected and refracted waves. This also occurs with light and this makes objects you see across an interface appear to be shifted relative to where they really are. For example, if you look straight down at an object at the bottom of a glass of water, it looks closer than it really is. A good way to visualize how light and sound refract is to shine a flashlight into a bowl of slightly cloudy water noting the refraction angle with respect to the incidence angle.

Refraction takes place at an interface due to the different velocities of the acoustic waves within the two materials. The velocity of sound in each material is determined by the material properties (elastic modules and density) for that material. In the animation below, a series of plane waves are shown traveling in one material and entering a second material that has a higher acoustic velocity. Therefore, when the wave encounters the interface between these two materials, the portion of the wave in the second material is moving faster than the portion of the wave in the first material. It can be seen that this causes the wave to bend.

Snell's Law describes the relationship between the angles and the velocities of the waves. Snell's law equates the ratio of material velocities **v1** and **v2** to the ratio of the **sine's** of incident (θ_1) and refraction (θ_2) angles, as shown in the following equation.

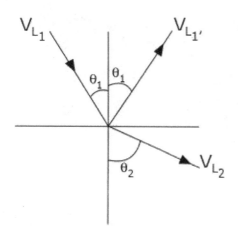

$$\frac{\text{sine}_1}{V_{L_1}} = \frac{\text{sine}_2}{V_{L_2}}$$

Where:

V_{L1} is the longitudinal wave velocity in material 1.

V_{L2} is the longitudinal wave velocity in material 2.

Note that in the diagram, there is a reflected longitudinal wave (V_{L1}) shown. This wave is reflected at the same angle as the incident wave because the two waves are traveling in the same material and, therefore, have the same velocities. This reflected wave is unimportant in our explanation of Snell's Law, but it should be remembered that some of the wave energy is reflected at the interface.

Piezoelectric Transducers

The conversion of electrical pulses to mechanical vibrations and the conversion of returned mechanical vibrations back into electrical energy is the basis for ultrasonic testing. The active element is the heart of the transducer as it converts the electrical energy to acoustic energy, and vice versa. The active element is basically a piece polarized material (i.e. some parts of the molecule are positively charged, while other parts of the molecule are negatively charged) with electrodes attached to two of its opposite faces. When an electric field is applied across the material, the polarized molecules will align themselves with the electric field, resulting in induced dipoles within the molecular or crystal structure of the material. This alignment of molecules will cause the material to change dimensions. This phenomenon is known as electrostriction. In addition, a permanently-polarized material such as quartz ($SiO2$) or barium titanate ($BaTiO3$) will produce an electric field when the material changes dimensions as a result of an imposed mechanical force. This phenomenon is known as the piezoelectric effect.

The thickness of the active element is determined by the desired frequency of the transducer. A thin wafer element vibrates with a wavelength that is twice its thickness. Therefore, piezoelectric crystals are cut to a thickness that is 1/2 the desired radiated wavelength. The higher the frequency of the transducer, the thinner the active element. The primary reason that high frequency contact transducers are not produced in because the element is very thin and too fragile.

Characteristics of Piezoelectric Transducers

The transducer is a very important part of the ultrasonic instrumentation system. As discussed on the previous page, the transducer incorporates a piezoelectric element, which converts electrical signals into mechanical vibrations (transmit mode) and mechanical vibrations into electrical signals (receive mode). Many factors, including material, mechanical and electrical construction, and the external mechanical and electrical load conditions, influence the behavior a transducer. Mechanical construction includes parameters such as radiation surface area, mechanical damping, housing, connector type and other variables of physical construction. As of this writing, transducer manufactures are hard pressed when constructing two transducers that have identical performance characteristics.

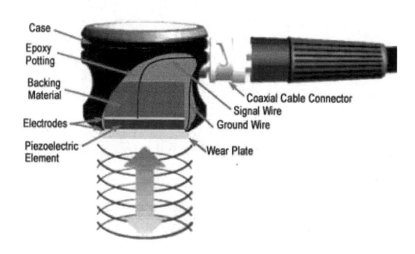

A cut away of a typical contact transducer is shown above. It was previously learned that the piezoelectric element is cut to 1/2 the desired wavelength. To get as much energy out of the transducer as possible, an impedance matching is placed between the active element and the face of the transducer. Optimal impedance matching is achieved by sizing the matching layer so that its thickness is 1/4 wavelength. This keeps waves that were reflected within the matching layer in phase when they exit the layer as illustrated in the image to the right. For contact transducers, the matching layer is made from a material that has an acoustical impedance between the active element and steel. Immersion transducers have a matching layer with an acoustical impedance between the active element and water. Contact transducers also often incorporate a wear plate to protect the matching layer and active element from scratch.

The backing material supporting the crystal has a great influence on damping characteristics of a transducer. Using a backing material with an impedance similar to that of the active element will produce the most effective damping. Such a transducer will have a narrow bandwidth resulting in higher sensitivity. As the mismatch in impedance between the active element and the backing material increases, material penetration increased but transducer sensitivity is reduced.

Transducer Efficiency, Bandwidth and Frequency

Some transducers are specially fabricated to be more efficient transmitters and others to be more efficient receivers. A transducer that performs well in one application will not always produce the desired results in a different application. For example, sensitivity to small defects is proportional to the product of the efficiency of the transducer as a transmitter and a receiver. Resolution, the ability to locate defects near surface or in close proximity in the material, requires a highly damped transducer.

It is also important to understand the concept of bandwidth, or range of frequencies, associated with a transducer. The frequency noted on a transducer is the central or center frequency and depends primarily on the backing material. Highly damped transducers will respond to frequencies above and below the central frequency. The broad frequency range provides a transducer with high resolving power. Less damped transducers will exhibit a narrower frequency range, poorer resolving power, but greater penetration.

Transducers are constructed to withstand some abuse, but they should be handled carefully. Misuse such as dropping can cause cracking of the wear plate, element, or the backing material. Damage to a transducer is often noted on the a-scan presentation as an enlargement of the initial pulse.

Transducer Beam Spread

Round transducers are often referred to as piston source transducers because the sound field resembles a cylindrical mass in front of the transducer. However, the energy in the beam does not remain in a cylinder, but instead spread out as it propagates through the material. The phenomenon is usually referred to as beam spread but is sometimes also called beam divergence or ultrasonic diffraction. Although beam spread must be considered when performing an ultrasonic inspection, it is important to note that in the far field, or Fraunhofer zone, the maximum sound pressure is always found along the acoustic axis (centerline) of the transducer. Therefore, the strongest reflection are likely to come from the area directly in front of the transducer.

Beam spread occurs because the vibrating particle of the material (through which the wave is traveling) do not always transfer all of their energy in the direction of wave propagation. Recall that waves propagate through that transfer of energy from one particle to another in the medium. If the particles are not directly aligned in the direction of wave propagation, some of the energy will get transferred off at an angle. (Picture what happens when one ball hits another second ball slightly off center). In the near field constructive and destructive wave interference fill the sound field with fluctuation. At the start of the far field, however, the beam strength is always greatest at the center of the beam and diminishes as it spreads outward.

Beam spread is greater when using a low frequency transducer than when using a high frequency transducer. As the diameter of the transducer increases the beam spread will be reduced.

Transducer Testing

As part of the documentation process, an extensive database containing records of the waveform and spectrum of each transducer is maintained and can be accessed for comparative or statistical studies of transducer characteristics.

Manufactures often provide time and frequency domain plots for each transducer. The signals below were generated by a spiked pulser. The waveform image on the left shows the test response signal in the time domain (amplitude versus time). The spectrum image on the right shows the same signal in the frequency domain (amplitude versus frequency). The signal path is usually a reflection from the back wall (fused silica) with the reflection in the far field of the transducer.

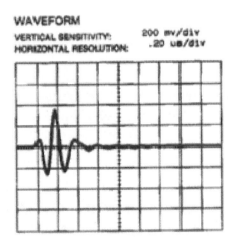 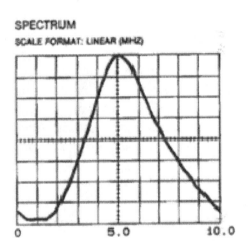

Other tests may include the following:

- **Electrical Impedance Plots** provide important information about the design and construction of a transducer and can allow users to obtain electrically similar transducers from multiple sources.
- **Beam Alignment Measurements** provide data on the degree of alignment between the sound beam axis and the transducer housing. This information is particularly useful in applications that require a high degree of certainty regarding beam positioning with respect to a mechanical reference surface.
- **Beam Profiles** provide valuable information about transducer sound field characteristics. Transverse beam profiles are created by scanning the transducer across a target (usually either a steel ball or rod) at a given distance from the transducer face and are used to determine focal spot size and beam symmetry. Axial beam profiles are created by recording the pulse-echo amplitude of the sound field as a function of distance from the transducer face and provide data on depth of field and focal length.

Axial resolution

The spatial resolution of ultrasound in the ultrasound beam direction, also known as the depth, linear, longitudinal and range resolution. The axial resolution is the minimum distance in the beam direction between two reflectors which can be identified as separate echoes. The axial resolution is slightly more than half the spatial pulse length, which is the number of waves in the transmitted ultrasound pulse (determined by the Q factor) multiplied by their wavelength (determined by the transducer frequency).

Digital scan converter

A component of all modern ultrasound imaging instruments that digitizes the scanned information and converts the ultrasound echoes into a two-dimensional B mode image composed of pixels. The digital scan converter is composed of an analogue to digital converter ADC, a computer and computer memory, and a digital to analogue converter DAC. In most ultrasound instruments, the ADC digitizes the echo amplitudes into 6 or 7 bits, i.e. 26 (64) or 27 (128) grey levels. The digital information is stored in the computer memory as a digital matrix, usually composed of $512 \cdot 512$ pixels. Each digitized echo is positioned in the matrix according to transducer or transducer element position (determining the horizontal pixel position), and to the time lapse from pulse transmission to echo detection (determining the vertical or depth position in the matrix). The DAC converts this true digital image into an analogue image on a TV monitor, by assigning each pixel in the analogue image a brightness determined by the digital number of the pixel in the digital image matrix.

Analogue-to-digital converter (ADC)

Electronic device which converts the analogue audiofrequency signals from, for example, an MR or ultrasound receiver into digital form so that it can be stored and processed by the computer. Important parameters for determining the performance of an ADC include the sampling speed and word length.

This Doppler effect in tissues maybe expressed as an equation as shown in this figure. Simply stated, the Doppler shift (Fd) of ultrasound will depend on both the transmitted frequency (fo) and the velocity (V) of the moving blood. This returned frequency is also called the "frequency shift" or "Doppler shift" and is highly dependent upon the angle (?) between the beam of ultrasound transmitted from the transducer and the moving red blood cells. The velocity of sound in blood is constant (c) and is an important part of the Doppler equation.

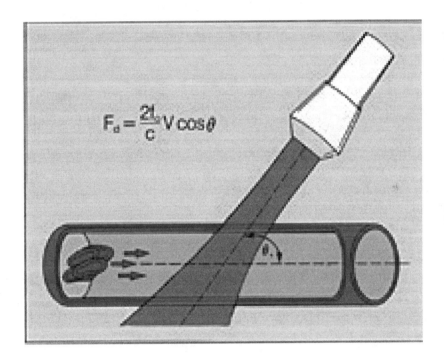

Doppler Key Points

Aliasing is an artifact that lowers the frequency components when the PRF is less than 2 times the highest frequency of a Doppler signal

Beat frequency, for CW Doppler, is the Doppler shift

Ensemble length -packet size, shots per line- is the number of pulses per scan line. In color Doppler, each line of sight most be pulsed several times

FFT. Fast Fourier Transform analyzer is a common device that performs spectral analysis in ultrasound instruments. In this case, it displays different quadrature Doppler frequencies, or reflector velocities when a sample volume cursor is used (Doppler frequency is proportional to reflector velocity) along time

High pass filter is the wall filter

Nyquist Frequency is the maximum frequency that can be sampled without aliasing. NF = PRF/2 (PRF stands for Pulse Repetition Frequency)

Quadrature detection is a signal processing method for directional Doppler in which the signal reference frequency for two channels differ in phase by 1/4 period. The output Doppler signal phase for both channels also depends on the Doppler shift, whether positive or negative

Spectral analysis is the quantitative analysis to display the distribution of frequencies

Variance is the variation of Doppler frequencies within each pixel during a pulse packet, effective to detect turbulence with color Doppler

The Doppler Principle

The Direction and Velocity of Flow

The fact that makes frequency of the Doppler effect more than just an interesting curiosity is that it actually provides a method that is used to measure the direction and speed of moving red blood cells. Clinically we are most interested in measuring velocity since, as mentioned above, it is altered in disease states.

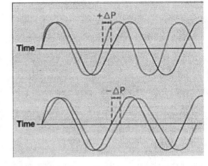

A Doppler system then compares the transmitted waveform with the received waveform for a change in frequency . These are called "phase shifts" and they are automatically determined within the Doppler instrument. If there is a higher returning frequency (+AP) then the flow is called a "positive Doppler shift" and represented as moving toward the transducer. If there is a lower returning frequency (-AP) then the flow is called a "negative Doppler shift" and represented as moving away from the transducer. All components of the Doppler equation, except velocity, are readily measured by the Doppler instrument.

The Doppler equation may be rearranged to solve for velocity of blood movement. The angle may be measured or may be assumed to be parallel depending upon orientation of the beam by the system operator.

$$V = \frac{c}{2f_o \cos\theta} F_d$$

The Doppler device can be regarded as a complex speedometer designed to detect red cell motion (i.e., blood flow) and measure its velocity. What is important to recognize is that:

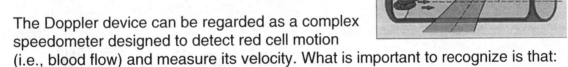

FREQUENCY SHIFT >>> DOPPLER EQUATION >>> VELOCITY DATA

The Doppler Display

All Doppler systems have audio outputs and listening to this is very helpful during a Doppler examination. The changing velocities (frequencies) are converted into audible sounds and, after some processing, are emitted from speakers placed within the machine.

High pitched sounds result from large Doppler shifts and indicate the presence of high velocities, while low pitched sounds result from lesser Doppler shifts. Flow direction information (relative to the transducer) is provided by a stereophonic audio output in which flow toward the transducer comes out of one speaker and flow away from the transducer.

The audio output also allows the operator to easily differentiate laminar from turbulent flow. Laminar flow produces a smooth, pleasant tone because of the uniform velocities. Turbulent flow, because of the presence of many different velocities, results in a commonly high-pitched and whistling or harsh and raspy sound.

The audio output remains an indispensable guide to the machine operator for achieving proper orientation of the ultrasound beam, even when Doppler echocardiography is being used in conjunction with an ultrasound imaging technique. The trained ear can readily appreciate minor changes in spectral composition more readily than the eye, given the same information displayed graphically. The major limitation of audio Doppler outputs is the requirements for subjective interpretation and the lack of a permanent objective record. The audio output from a Doppler machine is not the same as that received by a stethoscope or a phonocardiogram. The sounds detected with a stethoscope are transmitted vibrations or pressure waves from the heart and great vessels that are believed to be the result of rapid accelerations and decelerations of blood. The Doppler audio output, in contrast, is an audible display of the Doppler frequency shift spectrum produced by red cells moving in the path of the ultrasound beam. It is a sound produced by the Doppler machine that does not occur in nature and, therefore, it does not originate in the heart.

All newer generations of Doppler echocardiography equipment contain sophisticated sound frequency or velocity spectrum analyzers for hard copy recording. Most commercially available Doppler systems display a spectrum of the various velocities present at anytime and are, therefore, called "spectral velocity recordings.

Flow velocity toward the transducer is displayed as a positive, or upward, shift in velocities while flow velocity away from the transducer is displayed as a negative, or downward shift in velocities. Time is on the horizontal axis.

The internal working of such systems are complex but the results are rather simple. When flow is laminar and all the red cells are accelerating and decelerating at approximately the same velocities, a neat envelope of these similar velocities is recorded over time. When flow is turbulent, however, there are many different velocities detected at any one time (a wide spectrum of velocities). Such turbulence, produced by an obstruction to flow, results in the spectral broadening (display of velocities that are low, mid and high) and an increase in peak velocity as seen in disease states.

This display of the spectrum of the various velocities encountered by the Doppler beam is accomplished by very sophisticated microcomputers that are able to decode the returning complex Doppler signal and process it into its various velocity components. There are two basic methods for accomplishing this. The most popular is Fast Fourier Transform (FFT) and the other is called Chirp-Z Transform. These are simply ways for deciphering, analyzing and presenting vast amounts of returning data

The Effect of Angle

The Doppler equation also tells us that the angle the Doppler beam is relative to the lines of flow being evaluated is very important.

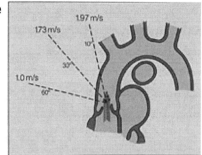

When the ultrasound beam is directed parallel to blood flow, angle Ø (cosine 0° = 1) and measured velocity on the recording will be true velocity. In contrast, with the ultrasound beam directed perpendicular to flow, angle Ø = 90 degrees (cosine 90° = 0) and measured velocity will be zero. Therefore, the smaller the angle, the closer angle cosine Ø is to 1.0 and the more reliable is the recorded Doppler velocity. A wider angle will result in a greater reduction in measured velocity compared to true velocity.

Thus, the more parallel to flow the Doppler ultrasound beam is directed the more faithfully the measured velocity will reflect true velocity. For practical purposes, angles of greater than 25° between the ultrasound beam and the blood flow being studied will generally yield clinically unacceptable qualitative estimates of velocity.

Color Flow Imaging In Clinical Practice

The Meaning of Color

The colors displayed on the flow map image contain useful information. By convention, Doppler color flow systems assign a given color to the direction of flow; red is flow toward, and blue is flow away from the transducer. Three typical color bars from a color flow imaging device are shown in the figure and give an initial frame of reference to the meaning of colors. Such color reference bars always appear on the screen of Doppler flow imaging devices. The center of the standard color bar on the left is black (white center reference mark) and represents zero flow.

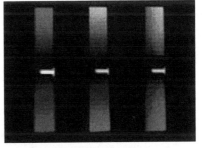

In addition to simple direction, velocity information is also displayed. Progressively increasing velocities are encoded in varying hues of either red or blue. The more dull the hue, the slower the velocity. The brighter the hue, the faster the relative velocity.

Color Flow Imaging In Clinical Practice
The Angiographic Concept

One way of conceptualizing Doppler color flow methods is to recognize its similarity to angiography. It provides a noninvasive "angiogram" of blood flow, where the contrast medium is the moving red blood cells and the detector of this contrast is ultrasound. The complex Doppler ultrasound processing circuitry allows for the detection of movement of these red cells in various directions - forward and backward through the heart. Doppler color flow information, however, is obtained and displayed in a cross-sectional image, making the spatial details of flow and anatomy readily recognizable. In effect, Doppler color flow looks inside the cineangiographic silhouette.

Creation of the Color Image
The Importance of Time

Time is the key factor to keep in mind. A conventional two-dimensional ultrasound imaging system is already working as hard as it can. Pulses must be transmitted along a given line, reflected from the heart valves and walls, then received. The process is repeated, line by line, through the entire sector arc that comprises several hundred lines. This completes one frame of information, usually in one-thirtieth of a second. In order to have the image appear as though it is continuously moving, the entire image must be updated 30 times in a second (30 frames/second). This results in relatively long waiting periods for the transmit-receive sequence to be completed. It also means that considerable amounts of information need to be quickly processed and presented in the image.

Creation of the Color Image

Expressed in its most simplistic terms, color flow systems add a separate processor that creates the color flow image based on the returning data and then integrates it with the two-dimensional anatomic image. Both the anatomic and the color flow data are then displayed in the final image.

The returning ultrasound data from any conventional scanner also contains frequency shift information that results from the encounter of the transmitted pulse with moving structures and blood. Until the advent of color flow imaging, this frequency shift data was simply ignored.

The key to color flow mapping is that the returning data may also be processed for the frequency shifts (or red blood cell velocities). Thus, color flow imaging systems take advantage of data that are available in every ultrasound image of the heart.

While this is a simplistic explanation, it is not true in most color flow systems. In reality, the lines of color flow data are alternated with lines of anatomic scan data. The anatomic data are acquired and received by conventional means and the color flow data are acquired, received, and processed separately.

Multigate Doppler

Doppler color flow instruments are all currently based upon pulsed wave (PW) Doppler methods. Conventional PW techniques are range gated. The Doppler sample volume is determined in range by the time it takes for the ultrasound pulse to travel to the area of interest and then back. If the same method was employed in color flow, it would simply take too long to sample over the entire image and there would be serious compromises made in frame rate.

Instead, all color flow systems are "multigated". This multigating takes advantage of Doppler information all along the line that is "ignored" in the conventional range-gated approach. In reality, each line has many gates that number in the hundreds.

It is best to think of the color flow map image as comprising little gates throughout the field of view, each gate containing some composite of the Doppler information. A typical image can consist of as many as 256 lines depending upon sector size and depth of range.

More About Color

All Doppler flow imaging systems encode the directions of flow into two primary colors: red and blue. Any number of color assignments could be made, but red and blue are chosen because they are primary colors of light (together with green).

here is also relative flow velocity information in the color hues; the brighter the color the higher the velocity detected. Thus, high velocities away from the transducer will appear as lighter shades of blue, and higher velocities toward the transducer will be represented by lighter shades of red, or even yellow. Low velocity flow will be represented by darker shades of these colors. Absence of flow is always represented by black.

Points of Discussion

Describe the relationship between ultrasound frequency and depth of penetration.

Ultrasound frequency is the number of cycles or waves of sound per second and is measured in Megahertz (MHz) or million hertz range. Higher frequency ultrasound provides greater detail, but has poorer penetration of tissues. This is because the small wavelengths allow for the differentiation of very small structures. Lower frequency ultrasound provides less detail but does have better penetration of tissues.

Medical ultrasound frequencies range from 3.5 to 7.5 MHz. For deep structures 3.5 MHz is appropriate. This is the frequency that is used the most for ER scans including the abdominal trauma exam. For thin patients and children, 5 MHz may be used which will provide more detail than 3.5 MHz as depth of penetration is not as important. 5 MHz is useful for testicular scans and transvaginal exams where detail is more important than depth of penetration. Frequencies of 7.5 MHz have a few specific uses. The high frequency gives great detail, but the depth of penetration is poor. 7.5 MHz is used primarily for foreign bodies, testicular, transvaginal and vascular scans since these are modalities where fine detail is more important than penetration depth.

Briefly describe the relationship between echogenicity and the depiction of ultrasound images as white, gray and black.

Echogenicity refers to the ability of a substance to reflect or transmit ultrasound waves.

An echogenic image is an image that is produced by an object that reflects most ultrasound waves. It will appear white on the ultrasound screen.

An anechoic image is one that is produced by an object that transmits most ultrasound waves. It will appear dark or black on the ultrasound screen.

An image that is gray is produced by an object that both reflects and transmits ultrasound waves to varying degrees.

What is the difference between a mechanical sector scanner and a linear electronic transducer?

In general, ultrasound devices all utilize a transducer. The transducer directs a narrow ultrasound beam along its line of sight, which returns a reflected ultrasound wave. This provides a one-dimensional line of information. By rapidly sweeping this line back and forth across a sector of tissue, a two-dimensional plane of information is generated, i.e., a cross-sectional ultrasound image of the tissue in question.

Mechanical sector scanners employ this principle by utilizing a small transducer element, which by rapidly pivoting back and forth (or through the use of a pivoting mirror), swings the ultrasound beam and generates a pie-shaped two-dimensional image. Since a single, small element is employed, these transducers are useful in situations where a narrow window is available, ie, imaging the heart through the space between two ribs.

As opposed to a singles winging beam, linear electronic (array) transducers utilize a linear arrangement (or array) of many small elements. When this device is held against the skin the elements fire rapidly in succession and in this fashion, generate a rectangular shaped two-dimensional image. Since many elements are required, linear arrays are longer (and more expensive) than mechanical sector scanners. In certain situations this can be a disadvantage. The advantage of linear arrays, however, lies in the fact that by providing small alterations in the sequence of firing of the individual elements, changes in the direction and depth of focus of the beam can be instantaneously achieved.

Discuss the conventional position of the marker on the transducer when scanning in the cross-sectional plane and describe the orientation of the resultant image on the display.

The cross-sectional or transverse ultrasound image should by convention, display the patient's right side of the body on the left side of the viewing monitor. The transverse ultrasound image is displayed so that the transverse "slice" is being viewed from the perspective of the patient's feet. (This is the same convention used for displaying CT images).

To produce a transverse image following this convention, the physician performing the exam should be on the patient's right side, and the transducer should be oriented in the transverse plane. The marker on the transducer should be directed towards the patient's right side. The resulting image will show a transverse view with the patient's right-sided structures (ie liver) on the left side of the monitor.

Define GAIN and TGC (Time Gain Compensator).

GAIN refers to the amplification of the received signal. It is the artificial increase in the strength of the signal. All parts of the image on the screen are equally affected (as opposed to TGC). Adjustments of gain should be done with respect to tissues of known echogenicity.

The TGC allows for 'fine tuning' of the attenuated signal. It allows one to sharpen the images of deeper is used when it is perceived that the gain in one part of the field is unequal to that of another.

Discuss the causes for the following common ultrasound artifacts:
- *pseudo-sludge (beam-width artifact)*
- *side lobe artifact*
- *reverberation artifact (ring down artifact)*
- *mirror effect*
- *gain artifact*
- *contact artifact*

a. Pseudo-sludge (beam-width artifact):

When the focal zone of the transducer is at the center of the gallbladder, the beam is of greater width at the posterior border of the gallbladder. The partial volume effect along the posterior wall results in the appearance of sludge (but it is really the posterior gallbladder wall). Also, gas bubbles in the duodenum can be projected adjacent to the gallbladder, simulating a gallstone.

b. Side lobe artifact:

This artifact is caused when weaker sound beams from the sides of the transducer are returned by a very reflective bowel-gas interface. This may appear as a line within the lumen of the gallbladder. To eliminate this artifact, try and alternate the angle of the transducer head.

c. Reverberation artifact:

This artifact is caused when ultrasound waves are being bounced back and forth between two or more highly reflective surfaces such as in the abdominal wall or a foreign body.

d. Mirror Effect:

Mirror effect is caused when the ultrasound beam is reflected back into the liver by the diaphragm and bounces back again to the transducer via the diaphragm. This results in intrahepatic structures appearing as if cephalad to the diaphragm.

e. Gain Artifacts:

Gain artifacts are caused by both overuse of gain in an attempt to enhance structures or under use of gain, which results in eliminating tissue character.

f. Contact Artifact:

When insufficient gel is used, the transducer makes only intermittent contact with the skin surface resulting in contact artifact.

6 Intensities:

Putting together spatial and temporal considerations we end up with 6 intensities:

- Spatial average-temporal average (SATA)
- Spatial peak-temporal average (SPTA)
- Spatial average-pulse average (SAPA)
- Spatial peak-pulse average (SPPA)
- Spatial average-temporal peak (SATP)
- Spatial peak-temporal peak (SPTP)

Since SATA averages both in space and time it's the lowest value. SPTP does not average --> highest value.

TIS/TIB/TIC

The **Soft Tissue Thermal Index (TIS)** is meant to be displayed for examinations in which the ultrasound beam travels a path which is made up principally of homogeneous soft tissue or a soft tissue/fluid path, as in a first trimester fetal examination or an abdominal examination. The **Bone Thermal Index (TIB)** is applicable to examinations in which bone is exposed to ultrasound, as could occur during Doppler blood flow examinations of a second or third trimester fetus. The **Cranial Bone Thermal Index (TIC)** pertains to examinations in which bone is at or very near the surface of the transducer, such as during transcranial, Doppler blood flow examinations.

ALARA principle of ultrasound exposure: **A**s **L**ow **A**s **R**easonably **A**chievable.

Key Organizations

American Institute of Ultrasound in Medicine
http://www.aium.org/

National Electrical Manufacturers Association
http://www.nema.org/

Key Exam Facts

- Ultrasound velocity is greatest in bone 4000 m/sec blood and muscle is about 1570 m/sec while fat is the slowest at about 1450 m/sec.

- The length of the fresnel zone increases when radius of transducer increases.

- Reverberation artifacts are caused by multiple reflections from interfaces.

- Doppler imaging in ultrasound detects change in frequency of sound.

- Speed of sound in a medium depends on the density of medium.

- Concerning Doppler studies change in frequency is related to blood flow.

- decibels are attenuated per cm for ultrasound in soft tissue.

- The amount of reflection at an interface is due to differences in acoustical impedance, and angle of incidence.

- Axial resolution (size in mm) in ultrasound is directly proportional to pulse length and constant with depth.

- Non specular reflections are those involving objects which are smaller than the ultrasound beam. The generally give weak signal since only a portion of the beam is reflected back towards transducer

- Concerning the thickness of the transducer used in ultrasound resonance occurs when the thickness is equal to 1/2 wavelength

- Q factor is calculated as operating frequency/bandwidth bandwidth is the range of frequency produces. We want the bandwidth to be small (ie a 3MHz transducer should only produce 3MHz sound). The more of other frequencies that are produced the lower the Q factor. The pure 3MHz is degraded.

- Lateral resolution depends upon the number of scan lines and the width of the ultrasound beam

- When a piezo electric crystal in an ultrasound transducer has a negative voltage induced in it, this is caused by dipoles.

- The TGC control in ultrasound compensates for differences in acoustical impedance.

- Aliasing in real-time ultrasound may be reduced by increasing the number of scan lines.

- The TGC is used in ultrasound to increase amplification of echoes at increased depths.

- A 5 MHz ultrasound beam passes from soft tissue to bone intensity is reduced significantly.

- Axial resolution in ultrasound is generally better than lateral resolution.

- Reverberation artifacts are caused by multiple reflections of same interface.

- The thickness of the transducer used in ultrasound are determined by thickness equal to 1/2 wavelength.

- Acoustic shadowing results when an ultrasound beam strikes a high attenuation.

- The amount of doppler shift is effect by turbulence, stenosis, and peak systolic.

- The lateral resolution in Ultrasound Imaging is determined by Beam Focusing and number of scan lines.

- The Doppler frequency increases when velocity increases, and greater transducer frequency.

- The critical angle in US refers to the angle at which all incident intensity is reflected.

- The 1/4 matching layer in ultrasound is used to increase the transmitted intensity into the patient.

- The following formula can be used to calculate Incident Beam after attenuation:
  $$dB = 10 \log I_1 / I_2$$

Secret Key #1 - Time is Your Greatest Enemy

Pace Yourself

Wear a watch. At the beginning of the test, check the time (or start a chronometer on your watch to count the minutes), and check the time after every few questions to make sure you are "on schedule."

If you are forced to speed up, do it efficiently. Usually one or more answer choices can be eliminated without too much difficulty. Above all, don't panic. Don't speed up and just begin guessing at random choices. By pacing yourself, and continually monitoring your progress against your watch, you will always know exactly how far ahead or behind you are with your available time. If you find that you are one minute behind on the test, don't skip one question without spending any time on it, just to catch back up. Take 15 fewer seconds on the next four questions, and after four questions you'll have caught back up. Once you catch back up, you can continue working each problem at your normal pace.

Furthermore, don't dwell on the problems that you were rushed on. If a problem was taking up too much time and you made a hurried guess, it must be difficult. The difficult questions are the ones you are most likely to miss anyway, so it isn't a big loss. It is better to end with more time than you need than to run out of time.

Lastly, sometimes it is beneficial to slow down if you are constantly getting ahead of time. You are always more likely to catch a careless mistake by working more slowly than quickly, and among very high-scoring test takers (those who are likely to have lots of time left over), careless errors affect the score more than mastery of material.

Secret Key #2 - Guessing is not Guesswork

You probably know that guessing is a good idea - unlike other standardized tests, there is no penalty for getting a wrong answer. Even if you have no idea about a question, you still have a 20-25% chance of getting it right.

Most test takers do not understand the impact that proper guessing can have on their score. Unless you score extremely high, guessing will significantly contribute to your final score.

Monkeys Take the Test

What most test takers don't realize is that to insure that 20-25% chance, you have to guess randomly. If you put 20 monkeys in a room to take this test, assuming they answered once per question and behaved themselves, on average they would get 20-25% of the questions correct. Put 20 test takers in the room, and the average will be much lower among guessed questions. Why?

1. The test writers intentionally writes deceptive answer choices that "look" right. A test taker has no idea about a question, so picks the "best looking" answer, which is often wrong. The monkey has no idea what looks good and what doesn't, so will consistently be lucky about 20-25% of the time.
2. Test takers will eliminate answer choices from the guessing pool based on a hunch or intuition. Simple but correct answers often get excluded, leaving a 0% chance of being correct. The monkey has no clue, and often gets lucky with the best choice.

This is why the process of elimination endorsed by most test courses is flawed and detrimental to your performance- test takers don't guess, they make an ignorant stab in the dark that is usually worse than random.

$5 Challenge

Let me introduce one of the most valuable ideas of this course- the $5 challenge:

You only mark your "best guess" if you are willing to bet $5 on it.
You only eliminate choices from guessing if you are willing to bet $5 on it.

Why $5? Five dollars is an amount of money that is small yet not insignificant, and can really add up fast (20 questions could cost you $100). Likewise, each answer choice on one question of the test will have a small impact on your overall score, but it can really add up to a lot of points in the end.

The process of elimination IS valuable. The following shows your chance of guessing it right:

If you eliminate wrong answer choices until only this many answer choices remain:	1	2	3
Chance of getting it correct:	100%	50%	33%

However, if you accidentally eliminate the right answer or go on a hunch for an incorrect answer, your chances drop dramatically: to 0%. By guessing among all the answer choices, you are GUARANTEED to have a shot at the right answer.

That's why the $5 test is so valuable- if you give up the advantage and safety of a pure guess, it had better be worth the risk.

What we still haven't covered is how to be sure that whatever guess you make is truly random. Here's the easiest way:

Always pick the first answer choice among those remaining.

Such a technique means that you have decided, **before you see a single test question**, exactly how you are going to guess- and since the order of choices tells you nothing about which one is correct, this guessing technique is perfectly random.

This section is not meant to scare you away from making educated guesses or eliminating choices- you just need to define when a choice is worth eliminating. The $5 test, along with a pre-defined random guessing strategy, is the best way to make sure you reap all of the benefits of guessing.

Secret Key #3 - Practice Smarter, Not Harder

Many test takers delay the test preparation process because they dread the awful amounts of practice time they think necessary to succeed on the test. We have refined an effective method that will take you only a fraction of the time.

There are a number of "obstacles" in your way to succeed. Among these are answering questions, finishing in time, and mastering test-taking strategies. All must be executed on the day of the test at peak performance, or your score will suffer. The test is a mental marathon that has a large impact on your future.

Just like a marathon runner, it is important to work your way up to the full challenge. So first you just worry about questions, and then time, and finally strategy:

Success Strategy

1. Find a good source for practice tests.
2. If you are willing to make a larger time investment, consider using more than one study guide- often the different approaches of multiple authors will help you "get" difficult concepts.
3. Take a practice test with no time constraints, with all study helps "open book." Take your time with questions and focus on applying strategies.
4. Take a practice test with time constraints, with all guides "open book."
5. Take a final practice test with no open material and time limits

If you have time to take more practice tests, just repeat step 5. By gradually exposing yourself to the full rigors of the test environment, you will condition your mind to the stress of test day and maximize your success.

Secret Key #4 - Prepare, Don't Procrastinate

Let me state an obvious fact: if you take the test three times, you will get three different scores. This is due to the way you feel on test day, the level of preparedness you have, and, despite the test writers' claims to the contrary, some tests WILL be easier for you than others.

Since your future depends so much on your score, you should maximize your chances of success. In order to maximize the likelihood of success, you've got to prepare in advance. This means taking practice tests and spending time learning the information and test taking strategies you will need to succeed.

Never take the test as a "practice" test, expecting that you can just take it again if you need to. Feel free to take sample tests on your own, but when you go to take the official test, be prepared, be focused, and do your best the first time!

Secret Key #5 - Test Yourself

Everyone knows that time is money. There is no need to spend too much of your time or too little of your time preparing for the test. You should only spend as much of your precious time preparing as is necessary for you to get the score you need.

Once you have taken a practice test under real conditions of time constraints, then you will know if you are ready for the test or not.

If you have scored extremely high the first time that you take the practice test, then there is not much point in spending countless hours studying. You are already there.

Benchmark your abilities by retaking practice tests and seeing how much you have improved. Once you score high enough to guarantee success, then you are ready.

If you have scored well below where you need, then knuckle down and begin studying in earnest. Check your improvement regularly through the use of practice tests under real conditions. Above all, don't worry, panic, or give up. The key is perseverance!

Then, when you go to take the test, remain confident and remember how well you did on the practice tests. If you can score high enough on a practice test, then you can do the same on the real thing.

General Strategies

The most important thing you can do is to ignore your fears and jump into the test immediately- do not be overwhelmed by any strange-sounding terms. You have to jump into the test like jumping into a pool- all at once is the easiest way.

Make Predictions

As you read and understand the question, try to guess what the answer will be. Remember that several of the answer choices are wrong, and once you begin reading them, your mind will immediately become cluttered with answer choices designed to throw you off. Your mind is typically the most focused immediately after you have read the question and digested its contents. If you can, try to predict what the correct answer will be. You may be surprised at what you can predict.

Quickly scan the choices and see if your prediction is in the listed answer choices. If it is, then you can be quite confident that you have the right answer. It still won't hurt to check the other answer choices, but most of the time, you've got it!

Answer the Question

It may seem obvious to only pick answer choices that answer the question, but the test writers can create some excellent answer choices that are wrong. Don't pick an answer just because it sounds right, or you believe it to be true. It MUST answer the question. Once you've made your selection, always go back and check it against the question and make sure that you didn't misread the question, and the answer choice does answer the question posed.

Benchmark

After you read the first answer choice, decide if you think it sounds correct or not. If it doesn't, move on to the next answer choice. If it does, mentally mark that answer choice. This doesn't mean that you've definitely selected it as your answer choice, it just means that it's the best you've seen thus far. Go ahead and read the next choice. If the next choice is worse than the one you've already selected, keep going to the next answer choice. If the next choice is better than the choice you've already selected, mentally mark the new answer choice as your best guess.

The first answer choice that you select becomes your standard. Every other answer choice must be benchmarked against that standard. That choice is correct until proven otherwise by another answer choice beating it out. Once you've decided that no other answer choice seems as good, do one final check to ensure that your

- 94 -

answer choice answers the question posed.

Valid Information

Don't discount any of the information provided in the question. Every piece of information may be necessary to determine the correct answer. None of the information in the question is there to throw you off (while the answer choices will certainly have information to throw you off). If two seemingly unrelated topics are discussed, don't ignore either. You can be confident there is a relationship, or it wouldn't be included in the question, and you are probably going to have to determine what is that relationship to find the answer.

Avoid "Fact Traps"

Don't get distracted by a choice that is factually true. Your search is for the answer that answers the question. Stay focused and don't fall for an answer that is true but incorrect. Always go back to the question and make sure you're choosing an answer that actually answers the question and is not just a true statement. An answer can be factually correct, but it MUST answer the question asked. Additionally, two answers can both be seemingly correct, so be sure to read all of the answer choices, and make sure that you get the one that BEST answers the question.

Milk the Question

Some of the questions may throw you completely off. They might deal with a subject you have not been exposed to, or one that you haven't reviewed in years. While your lack of knowledge about the subject will be a hindrance, the question itself can give you many clues that will help you find the correct answer. Read the question carefully and look for clues. Watch particularly for adjectives and nouns describing difficult terms or words that you don't recognize. Regardless of if you completely understand a word or not, replacing it with a synonym either provided or one you more familiar with may help you to understand what the questions are asking. Rather than wracking your mind about specific detailed information concerning a difficult term or word, try to use mental substitutes that are easier to understand.

The Trap of Familiarity

Don't just choose a word because you recognize it. On difficult questions, you may not recognize a number of words in the answer choices. The test writers don't put "make-believe" words on the test; so don't think that just because you only recognize all the words in one answer choice means that answer choice must be correct. If you only recognize words in one answer choice, then focus on that one. Is it correct? Try your best to determine if it is correct. If it is, that is great, but if it doesn't, eliminate it. Each word and answer choice you eliminate increases your chances of getting the question correct, even if you then have to guess among the unfamiliar choices.

Eliminate Answers

Eliminate choices as soon as you realize they are wrong. But be careful! Make sure you consider all of the possible answer choices. Just because one appears right, doesn't mean that the next one won't be even better! The test writers will usually put more than one good answer choice for every question, so read all of them. Don't worry if you are stuck between two that seem right. By getting down to just two remaining possible choices, your odds are now 50/50. Rather than wasting too much time, play the odds. You are guessing, but guessing wisely, because you've been able to knock out some of the answer choices that you know are wrong. If you are eliminating choices and realize that the last answer choice you are left with is also obviously wrong, don't panic. Start over and consider each choice again. There may easily be something that you missed the first time and will realize on the second pass.

Tough Questions

If you are stumped on a problem or it appears too hard or too difficult, don't waste time. Move on! Remember though, if you can quickly check for obviously incorrect answer choices, your chances of guessing correctly are greatly improved. Before you completely give up, at least try to knock out a couple of possible answers. Eliminate what you can and then guess at the remaining answer choices before moving on.

Brainstorm

If you get stuck on a difficult question, spend a few seconds quickly brainstorming. Run through the complete list of possible answer choices. Look at each choice and ask yourself, "Could this answer the question satisfactorily?" Go through each answer choice and consider it independently of the other. By systematically going through all possibilities, you may find something that you would otherwise overlook. Remember that when you get stuck, it's important to try to keep moving.

Read Carefully

Understand the problem. Read the question and answer choices carefully. Don't miss the question because you misread the terms. You have plenty of time to read each question thoroughly and make sure you understand what is being asked. Yet a happy medium must be attained, so don't waste too much time. You must read carefully, but efficiently.

Face Value

When in doubt, use common sense. Always accept the situation in the problem at face value. Don't read too much into it. These problems will not require you to make huge leaps of logic. The test writers aren't trying to throw you off with a cheap trick. If you have to go beyond creativity and make a leap of logic in order to have an answer choice answer the question, then you should look at the other answer choices. Don't overcomplicate the problem by creating theoretical relationships or explanations that will warp time or space. These are normal problems rooted in reality. It's just that the applicable relationship or explanation may not be readily apparent and you have to figure things out. Use your common sense to interpret anything that isn't clear.

Prefixes

If you're having trouble with a word in the question or answer choices, try dissecting it. Take advantage of every clue that the word might include. Prefixes and suffixes can be a huge help. Usually they allow you to determine a basic meaning. Pre- means before, post- means after, pro - is positive, de- is negative. From these prefixes and suffixes, you can get an idea of the general meaning of the word and try to put it into context. Beware though of any traps. Just because con is the opposite of pro, doesn't necessarily mean congress is the opposite of progress!

Hedge Phrases

Watch out for critical "hedge" phrases, such as likely, may, can, will often, sometimes, often, almost, mostly, usually, generally, rarely, sometimes. Question writers insert these hedge phrases to cover every possibility. Often an answer choice will be wrong simply because it leaves no room for exception. Avoid answer choices that have definitive words like "exactly," and "always".

Switchback Words

Stay alert for "switchbacks". These are the words and phrases frequently used to alert you to shifts in thought. The most common switchback word is "but". Others include although, however, nevertheless, on the other hand, even though, while, in spite of, despite, regardless of.

New Information

Correct answer choices will rarely have completely new information included. Answer choices typically are straightforward reflections of the material asked about and will directly relate to the question. If a new piece of information is included in an answer choice that doesn't even seem to relate to the topic being asked about, then that answer choice is likely incorrect. All of the information needed to answer the question is usually provided for you, and so you should not have to make guesses that are unsupported or choose answer choices that require unknown information that cannot be reasoned on its own.

Time Management

On technical questions, don't get lost on the technical terms. Don't spend too much time on any one question. If you don't know what a term means, then since you don't have a dictionary, odds are you aren't going to get much further. You should immediately recognize terms as whether or not you know them. If you don't, work with the other clues that you have, the other answer choices and terms provided, but don't waste too much time trying to figure out a difficult term.

Contextual Clues

Look for contextual clues. An answer can be right but not correct. The contextual clues will help you find the answer that is most right and is correct. Understand the context in which a phrase or statement is made. This will help you make important distinctions.

Don't Panic

Panicking will not answer any questions for you. Therefore, it isn't helpful. When you first see the question, if your mind goes blank, take a deep breath. Force yourself to mechanically go through the steps of solving the problem and using the strategies you've learned.

Pace Yourself

Don't get clock fever. It's easy to be overwhelmed when you're looking at a page full of questions, your mind is full of random thoughts and feeling confused, and the clock is ticking down faster than you would like. Calm down and maintain the pace that you have set for yourself. As long as you are on track by monitoring your pace, you are guaranteed to have enough time for yourself. When you get to the last few minutes of the test, it may seem like you won't have enough time left, but if you only have as many questions as you should have left at that point, then you're right on track!

Answer Selection

The best way to pick an answer choice is to eliminate all of those that are wrong, until only one is left and confirm that is the correct answer. Sometimes though, an answer choice may immediately look right. Be careful! Take a second to make sure that the other choices are not equally obvious. Don't make a hasty mistake. There are only two times that you should stop before checking other answers. First is when you are positive that the answer choice you have selected is correct. Second is when time is almost out and you have to make a quick guess!

Check Your Work

Since you will probably not know every term listed and the answer to every question, it is important that you get credit for the ones that you do know. Don't miss any questions through careless mistakes. If at all possible, try to take a second to look back over your answer selection and make sure you've selected the correct answer choice and haven't made a costly careless mistake (such as marking an answer choice that you didn't mean to mark). This quick double check should more than pay for itself in caught mistakes for the time it costs.

Beware of Directly Quoted Answers

Sometimes an answer choice will repeat word for word a portion of the question or reference section. However, beware of such exact duplication – it may be a trap! More than likely, the correct choice will paraphrase or summarize a point, rather than being exactly the same wording.

Slang

Scientific sounding answers are better than slang ones. An answer choice that begins "To compare the outcomes..." is much more likely to be correct than one that begins "Because some people insisted..."

Extreme Statements

Avoid wild answers that throw out highly controversial ideas that are proclaimed as established fact. An answer choice that states the "process should be used in certain situations, if..." is much more likely to be correct than one that states the "process should be discontinued completely." The first is a calm rational statement and doesn't even make a definitive, uncompromising stance, using a hedge word "if" to provide wiggle room, whereas the second choice is a radical idea and far more extreme.

Answer Choice Families

When you have two or more answer choices that are direct opposites or parallels, one of them is usually the correct answer. For instance, if one answer choice states "x increases" and another answer choice states "x decreases" or "y increases," then those two or three answer choices are very similar in construction and fall into the same family of answer choices. A family of answer choices is when two or three answer choices are very similar in construction, and yet often have a directly opposite meaning. Usually the correct answer choice will be in that family of answer choices. The "odd man out" or answer choice that doesn't seem to fit the parallel construction of the other answer choices is more likely to be incorrect.

Special Report: CPR Review/Cheat Sheet

1. Risk factors of stroke:
A: heart disease
B: high red blood cell count
C: TIA's

2. Signs of a stroke:
A: alteration in consciousness
B: sudden weakness or numbness in an extremity on one side of the body
C: sudden falls
D: unexplained dizziness
E: facial paralysis
F: difficulty speaking

3. Controllable risk factors of stroke and heart attacks:
A: high blood cholesterol
B: obesity
C: TIA's
D: smoking
E: heart disease

4. Chain of survival (adults)
A: early access (911)
B: early CPR
C: early defibrillation
D: early ACLS

5. Chain of survival (pediatric)
A: prevention of injuries and arrest
B: early CPR
C: early access (911)
D: advanced care

6. Rate of compression
A: adult-about 100x per minute
B: child-about 100x per minute
C: infant-at least 100x per minute

7. Depth of compression
A: adult- 1&1/2 to 2" compression (hands overlapping)
B: child- 1 to 1&1/2" compression (only heel of one hand)

C: infant- ½ to 1" compression or 1/3 to ½ the depth of infant's chest (2 fingers)

8. Ratio of compression to ventilations
A: adult- both one and two rescuers should use a 15:2 compression to ventilation rate
B: child- both one and two rescuers should use a 5:1 compression to ventilation rate
C: infant-both one and two rescuers should use a 5:1 compression to ventilation rate

9. Rescue breath with a pulse
A: adult-5 seconds (10-12 times per minute)
B: child- 3 seconds (about 20 times per minute)
C: infant- 3 seconds (about 20 times per minute)

10. Common causes of cardiac arrest in infants and children
A: breathing emergencies
B: onset following or from illness or injury
C: heart rhythm dysfunction

Adult one-rescuer CPR
1. establish unresponsiveness, activate EMS
2. open airway-look, listen, feel
3. if breathing is inadequate or absent give 2 slow breaths
4. check carotid pulse and signs of circulation in response to the 2 rescue breaths
5. if no pulse, give cycles of 15 chest compressions
6. after 4 cycles of 15:2 check pulse
7. if no pulse cont. beginning with chest compressions

**If victim begins breathing, place in recovery position.

Child one-rescuer CPR
1. establish unresponsiveness, send second rescuer for EMS activation if available
2. open airway-look, listen, feel
3. if breathing is inadequate or absent give 2 slow breaths
4. check carotid pulse and signs of circulation in response to the 2 rescue breaths
5. if no signs of circulation are present or heart rate is less than 60 bpm with signs of poor perfusion, begin cycles of 5 chest compressions and 1 breath
6. after about 1 minute, check signs of circulation. If alone, activate EMS, then continue compression/ventilation ratio
7. if signs of circulation are present but breathing is absent or inadequate, continue rescue breathing (1 breath every 3 sec. about 20 breaths per minute)

**If victim begins breathing, place in recovery position.

Infant one-rescuer CPR

1. establish unresponsiveness, send second rescuer for EMS activation if available
2. open airway-look, listen, feel
3. if breathing is inadequate or absent give 2 slow breaths
4. check brachial pulse and signs of circulation in response to the 2 rescue breaths
5. if no signs of circulation are present or heart rate is less than 60 bpm with signs of poor perfusion, begin cycles of 5 chest compressions and 1 breath, using 2 finger technique
6. after about 1 minute, check signs of circulation. If alone, activate EMS, then continue chest compression/ventilation ratio
7. if signs of circulation are present but breathing is absent or inadequate, continue rescue breathing (1 breath every 3 sec. about 20 breaths per minute)

**If victim begins breathing, place in recovery position.

Adult-Foreign Body Airway Obstruction-Unresponsive

1. establish unresponsiveness "Are you o.k?"
2. activate EMS
3. open airway and check breathing
4. attempt to ventilate
5. give up to 5 abdominal thrusts with victim on their back
6. open airway with tongue-jaw lift followed by a finger sweep
7. repeat steps 3 through til effective, then continue CPR as necessary

Adult-Foreign Body Airway Obstruction-Responsive

1. ask "Are you choking?"
2. give abdominal thrust (chest thrusts for pregnant or obese victim)
3. repeat cycle until object is cleared or victim becomes unresponsive
4. if victim becomes unresponsive-activate EMS
5. perform tongue-jaw lift followed by finger sweep
6. open airway and try to ventilate, if still obstructed, reposition head and try again
7. give 5 abdominal thrusts with victim on their back
8. repeat steps 5-7 til breathing is effective, then continue the steps of CPR as needed

Child-Foreign Body Airway Obstruction-Unresponsive

1. establish unresponsiveness "Are you o.k?"

2. activate EMS if a second rescuer is available
3. open airway and check for breathing
4. if breathing is absent or inadequate-attempt to ventilate, if unsuccessful reposition and reattempt
5. if ventilation is unsuccessful, perform 5 abdominal thrusts with the victim on their back
6. open airway with a tongue-jaw lift, and if you see the object, remove it-no blind sweeps
7. repeat steps 3-5 until ventilation is successful, then continue the steps of CPR as needed
8. if rescuer is alone and airway obstruction is not relieved after about 1 minute, active EMS

**If victim begins breathing, place in recovery position.

Child-Foreign Body Airway Obstruction-Responsive

1. ask "Are you choking?"
2. give abdominal thrust, avoid Xyphoid
3. repeat thrusts until object is expelled or victim becomes unresponsive
4. activate EMS if a second rescuer is available
5. open airway with tongue-jaw lift, if you see the object remove it, no blind sweeps
6. open airway , attempt rescue breathing, if no chest rise, reopen airway, and try to ventilate again
7. if ventilation is unsuccessful, provide 5 abdominal thrusts with victim on their back
8. repeat steps 5-7 til effective, then provide additional CPR if necessary
9. if rescuer is alone and airway obstruction is not relieved after about 1 minute, activate EMS

**If victim begins breathing, place in recovery position.

Special Report: Guidelines for Standard Precautions

Standard precautions are precautions taken to avoid contracting various diseases and preventing the spread of disease to those who have compromised immunity. Some of these diseases include human immunodeficiency virus (HIV), acquired immunodeficiency syndrome (AIDS), and hepatitis B (HBV). Universal precautions are needed since many diseases do not display signs or symptoms in their early stages. Universal precautions mean to treat all body fluids/ substances as if they were contaminated. These body fluids include but are not limited to the following blood, semen, vaginal secretions, breast milk, amniotic fluid, feces, urine, peritoneal fluid, synovial fluid, cerebrospinal fluid, secretions from the nasal and oral cavities, and lacrimal and sweat gland excretions. This means that universal precautions should be used with all patients.

1. A shield for the eyes and face must be used if there is a possibility of splashes from blood and body fluids.
2. If possibility of blood or body fluids being splashed on clothing, you must wear a plastic apron.
3. Gloves must be worn if you could possibly come in contact with blood or body fluids. They are also needed if you are going to touch something that may have come in contact with blood or body fluids.
4. Hands must be washed even if you were wearing gloves. Hands must be washed and gloves must be changed between patients. Wash hands with at a dime size amount of soap and warm water for about 30 seconds. Singing "Mary had a little lamb" is approximately 30 seconds.
5. Blood and body fluid spills must be cleansed and disinfected using a solution of one part bleach to 10 parts water or your hospital's accepted method.
6. Used needles must be separated from clean needles. Throw both the needle and the syringe away in the sharps' container. The sharps' container is made of puncture proof material.
7. Take extra care in performing high-risk activities that include puncturing the skin and cutting the skin.

Special precautions must be taken to dispose of biomedical waste. Biomedical waste includes but is not limited to the following: laboratory waste, pathology waste, liquid waste from suction, all sharp object, bladder catheters, chest tubes, IV tubes, and drainage containers. Biomedical waste is removed from a facility by trained biomedical waste disposers. The health care professional is legally and ethically responsible for adhering to universal precautions. They may prevent you from contracting a fatal disease or from a patient contracting a disease from you that could be deadly.

Special Report: What is Test Anxiety and How to Overcome It?

The very nature of tests caters to some level of anxiety, nervousness or tension, just as we feel for any important event that occurs in our lives. A little bit of anxiety or nervousness can be a good thing. It helps us with motivation, and makes achievement just that much sweeter. However, too much anxiety can be a problem; especially if it hinders our ability to function and perform.

"Test anxiety," is the term that refers to the emotional reactions that some test-takers experience when faced with a test or exam. Having a fear of testing and exams is based upon a rational fear, since the test-taker's performance can shape the course of an academic career. Nevertheless, experiencing excessive fear of examinations will only interfere with the test-takers ability to perform, and his/her chances to be successful.

There are a large variety of causes that can contribute to the development and sensation of test anxiety. These include, but are not limited to lack of performance and worrying about issues surrounding the test.

Lack of Preparation

Lack of preparation can be identified by the following behaviors or situations:

Not scheduling enough time to study, and therefore cramming the night before the test or exam
Managing time poorly, to create the sensation that there is not enough time to do everything
Failing to organize the text information in advance, so that the study material consists of the entire text and not simply the pertinent information
Poor overall studying habits

Worrying, on the other hand, can be related to both the test taker, or many other factors around him/her that will be affected by the results of the test. These include worrying about:

Previous performances on similar exams, or exams in general
How friends and other students are achieving
The negative consequences that will result from a poor grade or failure

There are three primary elements to test anxiety. Physical components, which involve the same typical bodily reactions as those to acute anxiety (to be discussed below). Emotional factors have to do with fear or panic. Mental or cognitive issues concerning attention spans and memory abilities.

Physical Signals

There are many different symptoms of test anxiety, and these are not limited to mental and emotional strain. Frequently there are a range of physical signals that will let a test taker know that he/she is suffering from test anxiety. These bodily changes can include the following:

Perspiring
Sweaty palms
Wet, trembling hands
Nausea
Dry mouth
A knot in the stomach
Headache
Faintness
Muscle tension
Aching shoulders, back and neck
Rapid heart beat
Feeling too hot/cold

To recognize the sensation of test anxiety, a test-taker should monitor him/herself for the following sensations:

The physical distress symptoms as listed above
Emotional sensitivity, expressing emotional feelings such as the need to cry or laugh too much, or a sensation of anger or helplessness
A decreased ability to think, causing the test-taker to blank out or have racing thoughts that are hard to organize or control.

Though most students will feel some level of anxiety when faced with a test or exam, the majority can cope with that anxiety and maintain it at a manageable level. However, those who cannot are faced with a very real and very serious condition, which can and should be controlled for the immeasurable benefit of this sufferer.

Naturally, these sensations lead to negative results for the testing experience. The most common effects of test anxiety have to do with nervousness and mental blocking.

Nervousness

Nervousness can appear in several different levels:

The test-taker's difficulty, or even inability to read and understand the questions on the test

The difficulty or inability to organize thoughts to a coherent form

The difficulty or inability to recall key words and concepts relating to the testing questions (especially essays)

The receipt of poor grades on a test, though the test material was well known by the test taker

Conversely, a person may also experience mental blocking, which involves:

Blanking out on test questions

Only remembering the correct answers to the questions when the test has already finished.

Fortunately for test anxiety sufferers, beating these feelings, to a large degree, has to do with proper preparation. When a test taker has a feeling of preparedness, then anxiety will be dramatically lessened.

The first step to resolving anxiety issues is to distinguish which of the two types of anxiety are being suffered. If the anxiety is a direct result of a lack of preparation, this should be considered a normal reaction, and the anxiety level (as opposed to the test results) shouldn't be anything to worry about. However, if, when adequately prepared, the test-taker still panics, blanks out, or seems to overreact, this is not a fully rational reaction. While this can be considered normal too, there are many ways to combat and overcome these effects.

Remember that anxiety cannot be entirely eliminated, however, there are ways to minimize it, to make the anxiety easier to manage. Preparation is one of the best ways to minimize test anxiety. Therefore the following techniques are wise in order to best fight off any anxiety that may want to build.

To begin with, try to avoid cramming before a test, whenever it is possible. By trying to memorize an entire term's worth of information in one day, you'll be shocking your system, and not giving yourself a very good chance to absorb the information. This is an easy path to anxiety, so for those who suffer from test anxiety, cramming should not even be considered an option.

Instead of cramming, work throughout the semester to combine all of the material which is presented throughout the semester, and work on it gradually as the course goes by, making sure to master the main concepts first, leaving minor details for a week or so before the test.

To study for the upcoming exam, be sure to pose questions that may be on the examination, to gauge the ability to answer them by integrating the ideas from your texts, notes and lectures, as well as any supplementary readings.

If it is truly impossible to cover all of the information that was covered in that particular term, concentrate on the most important portions, that can be covered very well. Learn these concepts as best as possible, so that when the test comes, a goal can be made to use these concepts as presentations of your knowledge.

In addition to study habits, changes in attitude are critical to beating a struggle with test anxiety. In fact, an improvement of the perspective over the entire test-taking experience can actually help a test taker to enjoy studying and therefore improve the overall experience. Be certain not to overemphasize the significance of the grade - know that the result of the test is neither a reflection of self worth, nor is it a measure of intelligence; one grade will not predict a person's future success.

To improve an overall testing outlook, the following steps should be tried:

Keeping in mind that the most reasonable expectation for taking a test is to expect to try to demonstrate as much of what you know as you possibly can. Reminding ourselves that a test is only one test; this is not the only one, and there will be others.
The thought of thinking of oneself in an irrational, all-or-nothing term should be avoided at all costs.
A reward should be designated for after the test, so there's something to look forward to. Whether it be going to a movie, going out to eat, or simply visiting friends, schedule it in advance, and do it no matter what result is expected on the exam.

Test-takers should also keep in mind that the basics are some of the most important things, even beyond anti-anxiety techniques and studying. Never neglect the basic social, emotional and biological needs, in order to try to absorb information. In order to best achieve, these three factors must be held as just as important as the studying itself.

Study Steps

Remember the following important steps for studying:

Maintain healthy nutrition and exercise habits. Continue both your recreational activities and social pass times. These both contribute to your physical and emotional well being.
Be certain to get a good amount of sleep, especially the night before the test, because when you're overtired you are not able to perform to the best of your best ability.
Keep the studying pace to a moderate level by taking breaks when they are needed, and varying the work whenever possible, to keep the mind fresh instead of getting bored.
When enough studying has been done that all the material that can be learned has been learned, and the test taker is prepared for the test, stop studying and do something relaxing such as listening to music, watching a movie, or taking a warm bubble bath.

There are also many other techniques to minimize the uneasiness or apprehension that is experienced along with test anxiety before, during, or even after the examination. In fact, there are a great deal of things that can be done to stop anxiety from interfering with lifestyle and performance. Again, remember that anxiety will not be eliminated entirely, and it shouldn't be. Otherwise that "up" feeling for exams would not exist, and most of us depend on that sensation to perform better than usual. However, this anxiety has to be at a level that is manageable.

Of course, as we have just discussed, being prepared for the exam is half the battle right away. Attending all classes, finding out what knowledge will be expected on the exam, and knowing the exam schedules are easy steps to lowering anxiety. Keeping up with work will remove the need to cram, and efficient study habits will eliminate wasted time. Studying should be done in an ideal location for concentration, so that it is simple to become interested in the material and give it complete attention. A method such as SQ3R (Survey, Question, Read, Recite, Review) is a wonderful key to follow to make sure that the study habits are as effective as possible, especially in the case of learning from a textbook. Flashcards are great techniques for memorization. Learning to take good notes will mean that notes will be full of useful information, so that less sifting will need to be done to seek out what is pertinent for studying. Reviewing notes after class and then again on occasion will keep the information fresh in the mind. From notes that have been taken summary sheets and outlines can be made for simpler reviewing.

A study group can also be a very motivational and helpful place to study, as there will be a sharing of ideas, all of the minds can work together, to make sure that everyone understands, and the studying will be made more interesting because it will be a social occasion.

Basically, though, as long as the test-taker remains organized and self confident, with efficient study habits, less time will need to be spent studying, and higher grades will be achieved.

To become self confident, there are many useful steps. The first of these is "self talk." It has been shown through extensive research, that self-talk for students who suffer from test anxiety, should be well monitored, in order to make sure that it contributes to self confidence as opposed to sinking the student. Frequently the self talk of test-anxious students is negative or self-defeating, thinking that everyone else is smarter and faster, that they always mess up, and that if they don't do well, they'll fail the entire course. It is important to decreasing anxiety that awareness is made of self talk. Try writing any negative self thoughts and then disputing them with a positive statement instead. Begin self-encouragement as though it was a friend speaking. Repeat positive statements to help reprogram the mind to believing in successes instead of failures.

Helpful Techniques

Other extremely helpful techniques include:

Self-visualization of doing well and reaching goals
While aiming for an "A" level of understanding, don't try to "overprotect" by setting your expectations lower. This will only convince the mind to stop studying in order to meet the lower expectations.
Don't make comparisons with the results or habits of other students. These are individual factors, and different things work for different people, causing different results.
Strive to become an expert in learning what works well, and what can be done in order to improve. Consider collecting this data in a journal.
Create rewards for after studying instead of doing things before studying that will only turn into avoidance behaviors.
Make a practice of relaxing - by using methods such as progressive relaxation, self-hypnosis, guided imagery, etc - in order to make relaxation an automatic sensation.
Work on creating a state of relaxed concentration so that concentrating will take on the focus of the mind, so that none will be wasted on worrying.
Take good care of the physical self by eating well and getting enough sleep.

Plan in time for exercise and stick to this plan.

Beyond these techniques, there are other methods to be used before, during and after the test that will help the test-taker perform well in addition to overcoming anxiety.

Before the exam comes the academic preparation. This involves establishing a study schedule and beginning at least one week before the actual date of the test. By doing this, the anxiety of not having enough time to study for the test will be automatically eliminated. Moreover, this will make the studying a much more effective experience, ensuring that the learning will be an easier process. This relieves much undue pressure on the test-taker.

Summary sheets, note cards, and flash cards with the main concepts and examples of these main concepts should be prepared in advance of the actual studying time. A topic should never be eliminated from this process. By omitting a topic because it isn't expected to be on the test is only setting up the test-taker for anxiety should it actually appear on the exam. Utilize the course syllabus for laying out the topics that should be studied. Carefully go over the notes that were made in class, paying special attention to any of the issues that the professor took special care to emphasize while lecturing in class. In the textbooks, use the chapter review, or if possible, the chapter tests, to begin your review.

It may even be possible to ask the instructor what information will be covered on the exam, or what the format of the exam will be (for example, multiple choice, essay, free form, true-false). Additionally, see if it is possible to find out how many questions will be on the test. If a review sheet or sample test has been offered by the professor, make good use of it, above anything else, for the preparation for the test. Another great resource for getting to know the examination is reviewing tests from previous semesters. Use these tests to review, and aim to achieve a 100% score on each of the possible topics. With a few exceptions, the goal that you set for yourself is the highest one that you will reach.

Take all of the questions that were assigned as homework, and rework them to any other possible course material. The more problems reworked, the more skill and confidence will form as a result. When forming the solution to a problem, write out each of the steps. Don't simply do head work. By doing as many steps on paper as possible, much clarification and therefore confidence will be formed. Do this with as many homework problems as possible, before checking the answers. By checking the answer after each problem, a reinforcement will exist, that will not be on the exam. Study situations should be as exam-like as possible, to prime the test-taker's system for the experience. By waiting to check the answers at the end, a psychological advantage will be formed, to decrease the stress factor.

Another fantastic reason for not cramming is the avoidance of confusion in concepts, especially when it comes to mathematics. 8-10 hours of study will become one hundred percent more effective if it is spread out over a week or at least several days, instead of doing it all in one sitting. Recognize that the human brain requires time in order to assimilate new material, so frequent breaks and a span of study time over several days will be much more beneficial.

Additionally, don't study right up until the point of the exam. Studying should stop a minimum of one hour before the exam begins. This allows the brain to rest and put things in their proper order. This will also provide the time to become as relaxed as possible when going into the examination room. The test-taker will also have time to eat well and eat sensibly. Know that the brain needs food as much as the rest of the body. With enough food and enough sleep, as well as a relaxed attitude, the body and the mind are primed for success.

Avoid any anxious classmates who are talking about the exam. These students only spread anxiety, and are not worth sharing the anxious sentimentalities.

Before the test also involves creating a positive attitude, so mental preparation should also be a point of concentration. There are many keys to creating a positive attitude. Should fears become rushing in, make a visualization of taking the exam, doing well, and seeing an A written on the paper. Write out a list of affirmations that will bring a feeling of confidence, such as "I am doing well in my English class," "I studied well and know my material," "I enjoy this class." Even if the affirmations aren't believed at first, it sends a positive message to the subconscious which will result in an alteration of the overall belief system, which is the system that creates reality.

If a sensation of panic begins, work with the fear and imagine the very worst! Work through the entire scenario of not passing the test, failing the entire course, and dropping out of school, followed by not getting a job, and pushing a shopping cart through the dark alley where you'll live. This will place things into perspective! Then, practice deep breathing and create a visualization of the opposite situation - achieving an "A" on the exam, passing the entire course, receiving the degree at a graduation ceremony.

On the day of the test, there are many things to be done to ensure the best results, as well as the most calm outlook. The following stages are suggested in order to maximize test-taking potential:

Begin the examination day with a moderate breakfast, and avoid any coffee or beverages with caffeine if the test taker is prone to jitters. Even people who are used to managing caffeine can feel jittery or light-headed when it is taken on a test day.

Attempt to do something that is relaxing before the examination begins. As last minute cramming clouds the mastering of overall concepts, it is better to use this time to create a calming outlook.

Be certain to arrive at the test location well in advance, in order to provide time to select a location that is away from doors, windows and other distractions, as well as giving enough time to relax before the test begins.

Keep away from anxiety generating classmates who will upset the sensation of stability and relaxation that is being attempted before the exam.

Should the waiting period before the exam begins cause anxiety, create a self-distraction by reading a light magazine or something else that is relaxing and simple.

During the exam itself, read the entire exam from beginning to end, and find out how much time should be allotted to each individual problem. Once writing the exam, should more time be taken for a problem, it should be abandoned, in order to begin another problem. If there is time at the end, the unfinished problem can always be returned to and completed.

Read the instructions very carefully - twice - so that unpleasant surprises won't follow during or after the exam has ended.

When writing the exam, pretend that the situation is actually simply the completion of homework within a library, or at home. This will assist in forming a relaxed atmosphere, and will allow the brain extra focus for the complex thinking function.

Begin the exam with all of the questions with which the most confidence is felt. This will build the confidence level regarding the entire exam and will begin a quality momentum. This will also create encouragement for trying the problems where uncertainty resides.

Going with the "gut instinct" is always the way to go when solving a problem. Second guessing should be avoided at all costs. Have confidence in the ability to do well.

For essay questions, create an outline in advance that will keep the mind organized and make certain that all of the points are remembered. For multiple choice, read every answer, even if the correct one has been spotted - a better one may exist.

Continue at a pace that is reasonable and not rushed, in order to be able to work carefully. Provide enough time to go over the answers at the end, to check for small errors that can be corrected.

Should a feeling of panic begin, breathe deeply, and think of the feeling of the body releasing sand through its pores. Visualize a calm, peaceful place, and include all of the sights, sounds and sensations of this image. Continue the deep breathing, and take a few minutes to continue this with closed eyes. When all is well again, return to the test.

If a "blanking" occurs for a certain question, skip it and move on to the next question. There will be time to return to the other question later. Get everything done that can be done, first, to guarantee all the grades that can be compiled, and to build all of the confidence possible. Then return to the weaker questions to build the marks from there.

Remember, one's own reality can be created, so as long as the belief is there, success will follow. And remember: anxiety can happen later, right now, there's an exam to be written!

After the examination is complete, whether there is a feeling for a good grade or a bad grade, don't dwell on the exam, and be certain to follow through on the reward that was promised...and enjoy it! Don't dwell on any mistakes that have been made, as there is nothing that can be done at this point anyway.

Additionally, don't begin to study for the next test right away. Do something relaxing for a while, and let the mind relax and prepare itself to begin absorbing information again.

From the results of the exam - both the grade and the entire experience, be certain to learn from what has gone on. Perfect studying habits and work some more on confidence in order to make the next examination experience even better than the last one.

Learn to avoid places where openings occurred for laziness, procrastination and day dreaming.

Use the time between this exam and the next one to better learn to relax, even learning to relax on cue, so that any anxiety can be controlled during the next exam. Learn how to relax the body. Slouch in your chair if that helps. Tighten and then relax all of the different muscle groups, one group at a time, beginning with the feet and then working all the way up to the neck and face. This will ultimately relax the muscles more than they were to begin with. Learn how to breathe deeply and comfortably, and focus on this breathing going in and out as a relaxing thought. With every exhale, repeat the word "relax."

As common as test anxiety is, it is very possible to overcome it. Make yourself one of the test-takers who overcome this frustrating hindrance.

Special Report: Additional Bonus Material

Due to our efforts to try to keep this book to a manageable length, we've created a link that will give you access to all of your additional bonus material.

Please visit http://www.mometrix.com/bonus948/ardmsultraphy to access the information.